Health Economics

Health Economics

An Introduction

Alan L. Sorkin
Johns Hopkins University
and University of
Maryland-Baltimore County

Lexington Books
D.C. Heath and Company
Lexington, Massachusetts
Toronto   London

Library of Congress Cataloging in Publication Data

Sorkin, Alan L.
    Health economics.

    Includes bibliographical references and index.
    1. Medical economics. 2. Medical economics—United States. 3. Under-
developed areas—Medical care. I. Title. DNLM: 1. Developing countries.
2. Economics, Hospital—U.S. 3. Economics, Medical—U.S. 4. Public health
administration—U.S. W74 S714h
RA410.S64   338.4'7'3621   74-25059
ISBN 0-669-93393-7

Published simultaneously in Canada.

Printed in the United States of America.

International Standard Book Number: 0-669-93393-7

Library of Congress Catalog Card Number: 74-25059

Contents

List of Figures

List of Tables

Preface

Within the field of human resource economics, the study of the economics of health has advanced rapidly in recent years. The importance of a clear understanding of this subject has increased as the nation moves closer to adoption of a comprehensive health insurance program.

Although the number of students enrolled in health economics courses is larger than ever before, instructors have been handicapped by the lack of an up-to-date textbook. This volume is an attempt to meet such a need. It is written at a basic level, designed to meet the need of undergraduates as well as students enrolled in schools of public health and other medical institutions. While the primary emphasis of the book is on the economics of the health services industry in the United States, approximately one-fourth of the material focuses on health problems in developing countries. Students with a course in the principles of economics will find this book more readily understandable than those with no previous background; however, an effort is made to present basic economic concepts that are essential in order to understand some of the more difficult sections.

Chapter 1 focuses on the distinctive economic characteristics of the health service industry as well as recent trends in expenditures and costs of medical care services in the United States. The next chapter analyzes the demand for health services. Numerous empirical studies are summarized and evaluated. The third chapter is concerned with health manpower. The severity of the physician shortage and the utilization of health auxiliaries in both developed and developing countries are among the topics discussed. Chapter 4 focuses on hospital costs. The major reasons for the acceleration in hospital cost inflation are presented. The next chapter emphasizes cost-benefit and cost-effectiveness analysis. Examples are drawn from both developed and developing nations. Chapter 6 is concerned with the interrelationship between health, population, and economic development in poor countries. The following chapter examines the relationship between health and poverty. Special programs such as the federally funded Neighborhood Health Centers and health programs for American Indians are considered. The final chapter deals with health insurance. The private health insurance industry as well as proposals for public health insurance are discussed.

The author is grateful to the following authors, publishers, and journals for permission to quote copyrighted material: *International Journal of Health Services*; the Johns Hopkins Press for the Josiah Macy, Jr. Foundation, *Auxiliaries in Health Care: Programs in Developing Countries* by N.R.E. Fendall; the Johns Hopkins Press, *Empirical Studies in Health Economics* by Herbert E. Klarman (Ed.); the Overseas Development Council; the *New England Journal of Medicine*; the *Journal of Human Resources*; the American Medical Association;

the *Milbank Memorial Fund Quarterly*; the McGraw Hill Book Company; the Bureau of Public Health Economics; the University of Michigan, Ann Arbor; the J.B. Lippincott Company; and the *Annals of the American Academy of Political and Social Science.*

Rita Keintz, John Owen, David Salkever, Martin Sorkin and Carl Taylor read the entire manuscript. Their constructive comments were most welcome, but the author is solely responsible for any errors. Mrs. Peggy Bremer typed the several drafts of the manuscript in her usual excellent manner. The manuscript was edited by Mary DeVries and the index was prepared by William C. Kiessel. Finally this book is dedicated to my parents, who inculcated an appreciation of learning that shall always remain with me.

1 The Health Services Industry

This chapter focuses on a variety of topics, including health indices, the distinctive economic characteristics of the health services industry, trends in health services expenditures, and medical care price inflation in the United States.

In what way can the economist contribute to an understanding of the health services industry? This question has been discussed by Victor R. Fuchs:

When an economist enters an area such as health—which has its highly developed technology and specialized terminology—he is often likely to be irrelevant or wrong. What, then, is the justification for such an inquiry? The major one is the fact that the question of the contribution of health services is being asked and answered every day. It is being asked and answered implicitly every time consumers, hospitals, universities, business firms, foundations, government agencies, and legislative bodies make decisions concerning the volume of health services present and future. If economists can help to rationalize and make more explicit the decision-making process, can provide useful definitions, concepts and analytical tools, and can develop appropriate bodies of data and summary measures, they will be making their own contribution to health and to the economy.[1]

Health Services

Health services can be defined as services rendered by the following:[2]

1. *Labor:* personnel engaged in medical occupations, such as doctors, dentists, and nurses, plus other personnel working directly under their supervision, including practical nurses, orderlies, receptionists, and laboratory technicians.
2. *Physical capital:* the plant and equipment used by these personnel such as hospitals or x-ray machines.
3. *Intermediate goods and services:* for example, drugs, bandages, and purchased laundry services.

This definition corresponds roughly to that which economists consider the "health industry." Payment for labor, capital, and intermediate input is the basis for estimating "health expenditures."

Approximately two-thirds of the value of health services in the United States represents labor input; somewhat less than one-sixth represents input of physical

1

capital; and the remainder represents goods and services purchased from other industries. These figures are all rough estimates. Information about the volume and composition of health services must be derived from a variety of official and unofficial sources. No census of the health industry exists. As the importance of the health industry grows, it becomes more imperative for the government to develop a census of the health industry similar, for example, to the census of manufactures.

Health Indices

Although the health services industry can be considered in terms of the industry inputs, it is often appraised in terms of industry output. One measure of the output or effectiveness of the health industry is selected indicators of health levels such as mortality rates, either age-specific or age-adjusted. The advantage of utilizing death rates for this purpose is that they are determined objectively, and are readily available in considerable detail for most countries. Moreover, the quality of the data is sufficiently good to use for comparisons over time within a country and at a moment of time between nations.

Health experts rely heavily on mortality comparisons for making judgments about the relative health levels of various subpopulations such as different racial and ethnic groups in the United States, or of smokers versus nonsmokers, or low-income and high-income persons. A fairly recent survey of health in Israel concluded that: "The success of the whole system of medicine in Israel is best judged not by an individual inspection of buildings or asking the opinions of doctors and patients, but by an examination of the health statistics of the country. Infant mortality is about the same as in many European countries, and life expectancy is equal to, or better than most."[3]

Differences within the United States are still considerable. For example, in 1969 the infant mortality rate for blacks was more than 60 percent higher than for whites. Moreover, the age-adjusted death rate for those living in poverty areas of our central cities is at least 40 percent greater than for higher income residents.

Comparing the United States with other developed countries, the differences are even greater (see Table 1-1). For males 45 to 54 (the age group at which earnings are maximized), the United States has the highest death rate of any country in the Organization for Economic Cooperation and Development, and has a rate that is almost double that of some of the other member countries. Although the United States has the highest per capita income in the world, its infant mortality rate is much greater than that of a number of countries in Western Europe and Japan. Moreover, the difference between the infant mortality rate in the United States and nearly all of the countries enumerated in Table 1-1 *widened* between 1960 and 1970. These major differences in death rates may imply serious deficiencies in the United States health system.

Table 1-1
Death Rates in OECD Countries Relative to the United States Average, 1970

[handwritten annotation: index of others rel to U.S.]

Country	Infant Mortality	Mortality Males 45-54	Mortality Females 45-54
United States	100	100	100
Iceland	70	N.A.	N.A.
Netherlands	64	63	68
Norway	64	65	58
Sweden	56	56	66
Greece	149	55	59
Denmark	72	66	86
Canada	95	76	78
Switzerland	76	64	68
France	92	78	73
Italy	149	70	71
Belgium	104	N.A.	N.A.
United Kingdom	95	73	85
Spain	141	67	73
West Germany (including Berlin)	119	90	108
Luxembourg	126	93	83
Ireland	98	79	100
Austria	131	80	82
Japan	66	65	75
Portugal	293	62	65

[handwritten annotation above Infant Mortality column: Death 100,000]

Source: World Health Organization, *World Health Statistics Annual*, Vol. I, Vital Statistics and Causes of Death (Geneva, Switzerland: World Health Organization, 1973), pp. 10-14, 620-23.

In recent years there have been a number of suggestions for better health *[handwritten margin note: problem of a health index]* indices that combine morbidity and mortality data. One interesting approach suggested by B.S. Sanders consists of calculating years of "effective" life expectancy, based on mortality and morbidity rates.[4] This index measures the number of years that a person is expected to live and be well enough to fulfill a role appropriate to his sex and age. This approach avoids the problem of interpreting measures of disease prevalence by measuring the effects of disease rather than the existence of disease. The years deducted from life expectancy because of disability are adjusted by some percentage factor that represents the degree of disability. The determination of these percentage weights is one of the most difficult problems to be considered in constructing a health index.

Another general index of health has been proposed by C.L. Chiang.[5] This index is a weighted average of age-specific components derived from the death rate and a measure of average duration of illness within each age group during a year. The index results from consideration of probabilistic models of the frequency of illness, the duration of illness, and the monthly distribution of mortality during a given year. The author presents a detailed description of the models derived, but it is not clear how well they fit empirical data on illness. The accuracy of the model needs to be tested on the basis of different definitions of illness before this question can be settled.[6]

Distinctive Economic Characteristics of the Health Services Industry

The health industry has a number of special features that make it an exception to many economic propositions which are more closely associated with industries whose firms sell their goods in competitive markets. While a number of industries may exhibit one or more of these characteristics, each of them applies to the health industry.

Consumer Ignorance

Very few industries could be mentioned where the consumer is so dependent upon the producer for information concerning the quality of the product as in the health services industry. Generally, he is also heavily influenced by the provider's recommendation concerning the quantity of health services to be purchased. These professional judgments are primarily made independently of any financial or cost considerations.

One reason for consumer ignorance is the large element of uncertainty concerning the effect of health services on an individual. Moreover, since medical services are purchased infrequently, the consumer does not have the experience to make a rational judgment. Finally, the medical profession often does little to inform the consumer concerning the results of *alternative* courses of treatment.

Nonprofit Motive

For much of the health and medical care industry, the profit motive is not an adequate explanation of behavior. This is especially true of hospitals, the majority of which are not operated on a proprietary or profit-making basis. While physicians on the hospital's staff admit, treat, and discharge patients, a hospital's responsibility to the community for the amount and quality of services rendered is vested in a board of trustees. Practicing physicians cannot serve as members of the board. This results in a separation between authority and responsibility in the voluntary hospital's management. This, plus the absence of the profit motive, may lead to inefficiency in hospital operations.[7] Moreover, this situation may be reinforced by the absence of competitive pressures in the hospital industry as well as lack of good information on the part of the consumer.

Restrictions on Competition

In some industries, where consumer ignorance is important, an individual obtains some measure of protection through the competitive behavior of producers, as in the automotive repair industry. If the producers engage in vigorous competition with one another, some of them will make an effort to inform the consumer about the merits of their product or service as well as those of their competitors. In the case of physicians' services the reverse is true. First, restrictions of entry for physicians are accomplished through the medical profession's control of medical schools, licensing requirements, and hospital appointments. Advertising is prohibited and price competition is extremely limited. It is considered unethical for a physician to disparage the service rendered by one of his colleagues. These restrictions probably result in higher prices for medical care services and larger incomes for physicians than would occur if restrictions on competition were eliminated.

Large Component of Personal Service

As indicated earlier, approximately two-thirds of the value of medical care services is associated with labor inputs. Thus, most health and medical care embody a large element of personal service. This fact has important implications for an economy such as the United States where wage increases are usually associated with productivity gains. For example, hospitals that compete with other industries for some types of unskilled and semiskilled workers, have not been able to offset the same proportion of wage and salary increases with productivity gains. This has been one major factor causing the rapid relative rise in hospital costs.

The "Need" for Medical Care

An increasing number of people believe that health services should be distributed according to need rather than effective demand (i.e., willingness and ability to pay). Because of the great advances in scientific medicine, health and medical care are now often considered the fourth human necessity ranking after food, clothing, and shelter.[8] When need is the only criterion for obtaining health services, much of the payment for these services is by a third party (e.g., government). This means that the consumer has less incentive to make certain that the services rendered are really worth the cost. Moreover, the supply of health services is not unlimited. A particular health program may be justified not because it is necessary or good but because it constitutes a more efficient use of resources than some alternative program.

The Uneven and Unpredictable Incidence of Illness

It is possible on the basis of epidemiological studies to predict morbidity rates for a population or selected group. However, for an individual, illness is not predictable. This implies the desirability of pooling payments to meet the contingency of illness. Pooling has taken the form of prepayment because health services cannot be repossessed by the provider as would be possible if one purchased a tangible commodity.

Another distinction arises because some health and medical expenditures occur regularly whereas others are associated with illness, which is unpredictable. The cost of regular, expected services may be prepaid but cannot be insured; the cost of occasional, unexpected services can be both prepaid and insured.[9]

External Effects

The economist defines *external effects* as involving positive and negative results for others that are the consequences of one's own actions. For example, in the case of a communicable disease such as smallpox, provision of a vaccination yields a benefit considerably greater than the prevention of the disease in one individual. When the transmission of the disease is stopped, the benefit achieved is a sharply lower probability of infection for everyone in the community. In such a case the private marginal benefit resulting from a vaccination program is less than the social marginal benefit. This implies that consumers may not be willing to pay enough for the service to justify its production by private producers and its provision would only be realized through a government program. Moreover, even if consumers were willing to pay for the program it is likely that the only institution with the resources to organize a mass campaign is the central government.

Mixture of Consumption and Investment Elements

Some expenditures for health services are provided merely to reduce anxiety, pain, or suffering. These are considered *consumption expenditures*. However, health services, especially when provided to members of the labor force, may render the individual more productive. (See Chapter 6 for specific examples.) In a sense the benefits in increased output represent a return on the investment resulting from the expenditure on health services. This expenditure is considered an investment in human capital.[a] In practice it is difficult to separate out consumption and investment elements of health expenditures. (See Chapter 5 for a pioneering effort in this regard.)

Medical Services, Research, and
Education as Joint Products

One of the difficulties in determining the costs of various activities within a medical school is that medical service is frequently produced jointly with medical education and sometimes also with medical research. For example, Table 1-2 indicates the distribution of faculty time in pediatric departments of medical schools. Most experts believe that by conducting a good medical educational program, a hospital improves the quality of care given to its patients. The teaching environment and the presence of students encourages intellectual curiosity and stimulates practitioners to render high quality care.

The tradition of using the poor population for teaching purposes has created

Table 1-2
Allocation of Faculty Time in Pediatric Departments of Medical Schools (in Percent), 1966-67

Time Allocation	Public Schools	Private Schools
Teaching alone	8.3%	9.8%
Teaching with patient care	25.2	23.7
Teaching with research and patient care	8.2	8.4
Teaching with research	4.3	4.7
Research alone	16.4	15.5
Research with patient care	7.5	6.6
Patient care alone	9.9	10.9
Administration	20.2	20.4

Source: Computed from Rashi Fein and Gerald I. Weber, *Financing Medical Education: An Analysis of Alternative Policies and Mechanisms* (New York: McGraw Hill, © 1971), pp. 18-19.

---

[a]Any good or service that makes individuals more productive can be considered an investment in human capital. Expenditures for health services, education, and migration are all examples of investment in human capital.

a problem because prosperity and health insurance as well as federally funded programs such as Medicare and Medicaid have reduced the volume of patients unable to pay for medical care. Therefore, many teaching hospitals are now using paying patients for teaching purposes.

Expenditures for Health Services

By nearly every measure available, the health services industry has emerged as one of the largest and most important in the United States in terms of total costs, employment, and federal expenditures. The influence of this industry on our economic, social, and political institutions has increased concomitantly. Moreover, it has become the center of a major public policy controversy.

Total expenditures for health and medical care in fiscal year 1972-73 reached $94.1 billion or 7.7 percent of gross national product (GNP).[10] Only five years earlier the figure had been $53.1 billion or 6.5 percent of GNP. In 1950 expenditures were only 4.6 percent of GNP. Thus, in 23 years health care expenditures as a fraction of GNP have grown by 67 percent. The rate of increase in expenditures for medical care had slowed somewhat from 1970-74 because of the imposition of the wage-price freeze, but now that the freeze has been lifted expenditures are rising rapidly. (See Table 1-3.) Some experts expect that medical expenditures may reach 10 percent of GNP by 1980.

A variety of factors have accounted for the rapid growth in medical expenditures, including a continuous increase in the demand for health services, recently augmented by a sharp advance in government financing; new methods of paying for health care, including the continuous growth of insurance; and extraordinarily large and sustained increases in health care prices.[11]

From the end of World War II until 1966, public outlays were approximately 25 percent of total expenditures for health and medical care. Expenditures within both the public and private sectors were increasing rapidly, but at roughly the same rate. Within the public sector, state and local governments were actually spending more than the federal government. The implementation of several major health programs in 1966, particularly Medicare and Medicaid changed these relationships.[b] Public expenditures reached $37.6 billion in fiscal year 1973 and represented nearly 40 percent of the total. The federal government accounted for about two-thirds of all government expenditures for health and medical care in fiscal year 1973; the remainder was from state and local funds. This distribution has fluctuated only slightly in recent years, though in 1965, the year before Medicare and Medicaid were enacted, the federal share was less than half as great.

---

[b]These programs were incorporated in the Social Security Amendments of 1965. Medicare combines two programs of health insurance for persons 65 and over. Medicaid is a federal grant-in-aid medical assistance program operating through the states, intended to cover, by 1975, virtually all the medically needy.

Table 1-3

Expenditures for Health and Medical Care, Selected Fiscal Years, 1928-29 Through 1972-73 (Dollar Amounts in Millions)

Type of Expenditure	1928-29	1939-40	1949-50	1959-60	1969-70	1972-73
Total (dollars)	3,589.1	3,804.6	12,027.3	25,856.2	68,083.1	94,069.6
Private expenditures	3,112.0	3,023.0	8,962.0	19,461.0	42,851.0	56,516.0
Health and medical services[a]	3,010.0	2,992.0	8,747.0	18,937.0	40,685.0	53,773.0
Medical facilities construction	102.0	31.0	215.0	524.0	2,166.0	2,743.0
Public expenditures	477.1	781.6	3,065.3	6,395.2	25,232.1	37,553.6
Health and medical services	372.5	679.5	2,470.2	5,346.3	22,576.4	34,009.0
Medical research	– –	2.6	72.9	471.2	1,652.8	2,057.0
Medical facilities construction	104.7	99.6	522.3	577.7	1,003.0	1,487.6
Total expenditures as a percent of gross national product	3.6	4.0	4.6	5.2	7.1	7.7
Public expenditures as a percent of total expenditures	13.3	20.5	25.5	24.7	37.1	39.9
Personal care expenditures	3,165.2	3,501.8	10,400.4	22,728.7	59,126.7	80,048.0
Private expenditures	2,883.0	2,979.0	8,298.0	17.799.0	38,577.0	49,713.0
Public expenditures	282.0	522.8	2,102.4	4,929.7	20,549.7	30,335.0
Percent from private expenditures	91.1	85.1	79.8	78.3	65.2	62.1
Direct payments	88.5	82.8	68.3	55.5	39.4	35.1
Insurance benefits	– –	– –	8.5	20.7	24.4	25.6
Public expenditures	8.9	14.9	20.2	21.7	34.8	37.9

[a]Includes medical research.

Source: Alfred M. Skolnik and Sophie R. Dales, "Social Welfare Expenditures, 1972-1973," *Social Security Bulletin*, Vol. 37, No. 1, January 1974, p. 13.

In 1950 private health insurance was a $1.2 billion annual enterprise. In 1973 it accounted for $23.8 billion, with some $20.5 billion allocated for health services expenditures and the remainder for administration and overhead. (See Table 1-3.) Insurance accounted for about 41.2 percent of private personal care expenditures and 25.6 percent of total personal care expenditures.[12]

About 4.3 million persons were employed in the health services industry in 1970—in hospitals, clinics, doctor's offices, laboratories, with 63 percent of those working in hospitals.[13] This figure does not include more than a million persons employed in the manufacture and distribution of drugs, as well as several other occupations that are part of the larger health field. However, even with the restricted census definition of the health service industry, the medical care industry ranked as the second largest employer of manpower in 1970, exceeded only by construction. Between 1960 and 1970 the total number of employees working in the health services industry increased by 59 percent compared with a

54 percent increase between 1950 and 1960. The U.S. Bureau of Labor Statistics estimates that in 1975 there will be 5.4 million persons employed in health services.[14]

Costs

Swiftly rising costs have contributed to rising discontent concerning the effectiveness of the American health care system. For example, the operation of the Medicare program cost $9.5 billion in 1973, compared to $6.5 billion only four years earlier.[15] The cost increases associated with the Medicaid program have been even more dramatic.

The United States has experienced a tremendous increase in per capita demand for health care. Expenditures per capita rose from $84.49 in 1950, to $447.95 in 1973. Eliminating the influence of rising prices, it is found that the 1973 expenditures represented a 139 percent increase over 1950, an average annual increase of slightly less than 4 percent. Much of this growth has occurred in the past seven years.[c]

There are a number of reasons for increased demand in spite of sharply rising prices for medical care. Increased income is one factor, but the demand for health services has grown far more rapidly than could be explained by rising incomes. Other contributing factors include a relative increase in the number of older persons in the population; higher educational levels and concomitant greater health awareness; urbanization of the population; a relative increase in the number of health care providers so that patients have easier access to medical care; and the growth of insurance, prepayment, and other third party payments. However, as Herman M. Somers points out, "the single most important element has been the spectacular advance in medical terminology which within this century has revolutionized medical care from a service of generally dubious efficacy to one regarded as an essential service to which all individuals have a fundamental right to obtain."[16]

Fuchs has endeavored to explain the factors that have contributed to the growth in medical care expenditures from 1947-67.

As indicated in Table 1-4, nearly one-half of the average annual rate of change of medical care expenditures is accounted for by rising prices with growth of real national income per person accounting for only one-third.

Price Changes

In spite of the steady growth in the utilization of health services, price increases have been a major element in increasing costs. For example, from 1960-68

---

[c]Expenditures have been converted to the 1973 level of medical care prices, based on the medical care component of the consumer price index. Since medical care prices have been rising much faster than other prices, this figure understates the per capita increase in constant *general* dollars spent for health services. If the adjustment had been based on the overall consumer price index, rather than the medical care component, the increase from 1950 to 1973 would show 188 percent instead of 139 percent.

Table 1-4

Factors Contributing to Growth of Expenditures for Medical Care, 1947-67

Factor	Average Annual Rates of Change (%)		
	1947-67	1947-57	1957-67
Medical care expenditures accounted for by:			
Rise in price of medical care	3.7	3.7	3.6
Growth of population	1.6	1.8	1.5
Growth of real national income per capita	2.3	2.0	2.5
Decline in quantity demanded because of rise in relative price of medical care	−0.2	−0.2	−0.2
Unexplained residuum	0.6	0.2	1.0

Source: Victor R. Fuchs, "The Growing Demand for Medical Care," *The New England Journal of Medicine*, Vol. 279, No. 4, July 25, 1968, p. 190. Reprinted by permission of *The New England Journal of Medicine*.

hospital prices rose three times as rapidly as utilization.[17] From 1965-69 the price of physicians' services rose twice as rapidly as the number of physician visits.[18]

While it is true that consumer prices have generally been rising, the medical price index has increased much more rapidly. From 1945 to 1973 medical prices advanced 226 percent while the index of all prices advanced 146 percent. By far the major influence was hospital costs, which increased 933 percent, nearly seven times as fast as all prices and more than five times as fast as all *services* in the consumer price index.

From 1965 to 1970 medical prices advanced very rapidly. The implementation of the large Medicare and Medicaid programs, which increased the demand for health services without augmenting supply, undoubtedly were partially responsible, but they were not the basic influences. The causes of inflation in the medical care industry are more fundamental, and have preceded the advent of new programs. During 1960-65, when all services rose at a 2 percent annual rate, medical services advanced at a 3.1 percent rate, 55 percent faster. However, from 1965 to 1967 medical service prices rose at an average rate of 7 percent compared with only 4.1 percent for all services, a difference of 71 percent. Since 1970 the prices of medical services has risen at approximately the same rate as that for all services.[19] The implementation of the wage and price controls in 1971, which were not lifted from the health services industry until 1974, was an important factor in limiting the recent rise in the price of medical services.

Hospital room and service rates, which advanced an average of 6.3 percent per year from 1960 to 1965, jumped 9.4 percent in 1966 and then 19.1 percent in 1967. However, from 1967 to 1973 hospital charges rose only twice as fast as the rate of price increases for all services.

Some economists have argued that the medical care price index may overstate the rise in the real cost of health services. Thus, Anne A. Scitovsky undertook extensive research to test the criticism that the consumer price index overstates the true price increase because of failure to take account of improved effectiveness of a physician visit or a day in the hospital. If this criticism were correct, a more valid measure could be obtained by calculating changes in the total cost of treating specified episodes of illness. Scitovsky measured medical cost changes in terms of the average cost of treatment of five common conditions—acute appendicitis, maternity care, otitis media in children, cancer of the breast, and fracture of the forearm in children. Focusing on the 1951-65 period, she found that the cost of treatment, with one minor exception, had increased considerably more than the medical care price index. The price index had risen 57 percent while the median increase in the cost of treatment was 87 percent, ranging from 55 to 315 percent.[20] Thus, on the basis of her study there is certainly no evidence to suggest an upward bias in the medical care price index.

Causes of Medical Care Price Increases

There are a number of major factors associated with the increase in medical care prices. Wage increases, the expansion of medical insurance programs, the relative shortage of physicians, the implementation of new and more expensive medical techniques, have all played an important role.[21]

Although some categories of health personnel still receive relatively low wages, in general their earnings have improved substantially and this has been one factor causing significant increases in hospital costs. Medical care is a very labor-intensive industry. Therefore, when wages rise, prices will rise commensurately. Wage increases of nonprofessional health personnel have risen sharply in response to unionization or the threat of unionization. This type of inflation is known as *cost-push inflation* since it originates with the increased factor costs for the seller or provider of services.

Demand-pull inflation, which occurs when consumer willingness to purchase services is greater than the supply offered for sale at constant prices, is also important in explaining medical care price inflation. The growth of medical insurance and the rise in consumer incomes both have increased demand for health services more rapidly than supply.

Another source of higher medical care prices is the increased use of new technology and equipment. Moreover, there has been considerable duplication by medical facilities, chiefly by hospitals, in providing these new services. Most authorities believe that a 70 percent utilization rate is required to justify the purchase of sophisticated medical equipment such as, for example, the facilities associated with an intensive cardiac care medical team. Yet, many of these facilities operate at only 20 percent capacity. This obviously leads to substantial price increases for the consumer.[22]

Physician Fees and Income

In theory, the private practitioner has considerable freedom in determining his fee schedule. However, there are a number of factors that can strongly influence the price he has set for his services, such as cost of service rendered, patient's income, customary fees in the community, the prevalence of medical insurance in the community, and limitations under the law or under the rules of professional associations.[23]

Standardization of fees in a community has been furthered by the movement toward using relative value scales, which have been sponsored by a number of medical societies. Such scales assign specified weights to certain physician services on the basis of a consensus among physicians. Given the price of an office visit (one unit), the prices of all other services can be determined. For example, if the physician's usual charge for such a visit is $5, then a one-unit procedure costs $5. Thus, if a physical examination is assigned a weight of four units, the cost is $20.

The median net income of self-employed physicians (M.D.'s) totaled $45,193 in 1973, up 45 percent from 1967.[24] From 1967 to 1973 the "all items" Consumer Price Index (CPI) rose 37 percent and the physicians' fee component of the CPI 41 percent. Over the long run, physicians' incomes have increased at a faster rate than their fees.

The rise in physicians' net income derives partly from an advance in productivity, that is, by providing more services in the same or fewer hours of work per week. There are indications that most of the physician's productivity advance over the long run took the form of seeing more patients in the same amount of time. The shift from house to office and clinic visits, improvement in medical science, the utilization of more capital equipment and auxiliary personnel, and formation of group practices, have all contributed to higher physician productivity.

Another factor may be improvement in collection rates, which rose from 88 percent in 1947 to 92 percent in 1966. There is reason to believe that Medicare and Medicaid have raised this rate even further. In addition the incomes of physicians have increased since the implementation of Medicare because of the payment of customary charges under the program. Many physicians previously charged their aged patients on a sliding scale and thus were paid less than their customary charges.[d]

A final factor that is of major importance in explaining the rise in physician incomes is the "doctor shortage." (See Chapter 3 for a discussion of the magnitude of the doctor shortage.) In economic terms the phenomena of rapidly

[d]According to the Medicare law, doctors must be paid, or the beneficiary reimbursed, "customary" charges for each service—that is to be within the range of fees "prevailing" in the community for similarly situated doctors; and that the fee must not be more than the carrier (the private insurance company that acts as a paying agency for the government) would pay for its own policyholders.

rising prices is closely associated with an imbalance between supply and demand.

Methods of Paying Physicians

The fee-for-service method of paying physicians, in which the patient is charged for each service performed, is criticized because it encourages some physicians to provide excessive care. Moreover, outside of a group practice setting, the referral of a patient to another physician means the loss of a fee. This may tend to encourage some physicians to undertake procedures for which they may not be qualified in order to avoid referral.

There are two other principal methods by which physicians can be paid for their services. These are (a) capitation and (b) salary.

The *capitation method* stipulates that a physician is paid a certain amount depending upon the number of people he cares for rather than the quantity of services provided. Thus, there is no incentive to maximize the volume of care. While the fee-for-service doctor may hesitate to refer his patients for specialist consultations, the capitation doctor may make unnecessary referrals.[25]

In many respects the *salary method* of paying doctors is like the capitation method, in that the physician is awarded a fixed amount for a given period regardless of the volume of services rendered. Yet, it differs in one substantial respect: it is associated with some form of organized medical practice such as a clinic or hospital.

As for the quantity of services likely to follow from salary payment, there is obviously no built-in inducement to a high volume as with fee-for-service. Instead, the inducement to good performance depends upon the organized framework in which the doctor functions rather than the method of payment.

In a salaried medical organization with good personal interrelationships the physician has every reason to consult with colleagues in other specialties. Such a pattern also permits the physician to undertake postgraduate studies periodically, without loss of income.[26]

Health Insurance

The post-World War II development of fringe benefits through collective bargaining and the growth of union-management health and welfare funds have been major forces in the tremendous growth of voluntary health insurance in the United States. (See Table 1-5.) In addition, this phenomenon was given considerable impetus by the threat of President Truman's proposal for public national health insurance to meet the problem of lack of individual resources to meet health care costs. In 1970 about four-fifths of the population under age 65

Table 1-5
Private Health Insurance Coverage 1940-70

would be nice to see these converted to rates in order to eliminate impact of pop. growth.

Number of Persons (in Millions)

Year	Hospital Care	Surgical Services
1940	12.3	5.3
1945	32.1	12.9
1950	76.6	54.2
1955	105.5	88.9
1960	130.0	117.3
1965	153.1	140.5
1969	175.2	162.1
1970	181.6	167.8

Source: U.S. Department of Health, Education, and Welfare, *Medical Care Costs and Prices, 1972* (Washington, D.C.: U.S. Government Printing Office, 1972), p. 94.

had some form of private health insurance, but the amount and type of coverage is often limited.

About 17 percent of the civilian population under age 65 (representing some 31 million persons) was still without insurance in 1970. Disproportionate numbers of these were children and the poor. For example, in 1970 only 36.3 percent of the population with incomes under $3,000 had hospital insurance and only 34.8 percent of the population at that income level had surgical insurance— this compared with 92.3 percent of persons with hospital insurance and 90.7 percent with surgical insurance in the $10,000 and over income bracket.[27] Medicaid protection applied to about 9.5 million poor families by the end of 1970, and an additional 1.25 million poor, disabled, and blind. The percent of persons aged 65 and over who had private health insurance was generally much lower, largely because of their coverage under the Medicare program.

The Medicare program relieves insurance carriers of the almost prohibitive task of insuring the aged—a high-cost, low-income group. The inability of the insurance industry to reach remaining parts of the low-income population successfully continues to be an important problem, apparently not within the capacity of the industry itself to resolve satisfactorily. The most serious present challenge to health insurance is the provision of more comprehensive benefits, covering a large proportion of family medical care costs.

For a long time the health insurance industry has been criticized for aggravating cost inflation by its imbalance in benefit coverage, which was originally centered almost entirely on hospital care and contributed to inappropriate and expensive patterns of utilization. Since people were covered for expenses incurred in a hospital, but not for ambulatory care, a strong tendency developed for use of hospitals even when care of a less expensive kind was more appropriate. In spite of the development of policies designed to extend insurance to broader protection, the emphasis still remains on hospital care. While no specific data are available, it is probable that over 80 percent of all insurance benefits are paid for hospital-related care.[28]

Recently the criticism has broadened to focus on the general lack of comprehensiveness in the scope of benefits in most private health insurance. Perhaps three-fifths or more of personal health care costs are not covered by private insurance.[29] Although consumers have been rapidly increasing their expenditures for health insurance, the proportion of consumer medical expenses met by insurance has advanced at a very slow pace and appears to have approached a plateau at an unsatisfactory low level. From 1959 to 1973 the increase has averaged approximately one percentage point a year, and the figure is presently about 40 percent of consumer expenditures. Thus, it would require another 10 years before more than half of consumer expenditures would be covered, and many experts consider even that level inadequate.

The advent of Medicare has intensified the pressure on the private insurance industry to increase benefit levels. The benefits available to Medicare recipients are far more extensive than those currently available to most people with private insurance. Thus, the inadequacy of the latter becomes more obvious.

However, the insurance industry is also affected by medical price inflation. If carriers are to broaden the range of insurance benefits, they must raise premiums, in order to maintain profit levels. However, if charges must be increased 10 percent or more each year just to finance the same package of benefits, it becomes less feasible to raise premiums for enlarged benefits. In fact, there is evidence that some carriers are being forced to retreat; deductibles and coinsurance that add to consumers' out-of-pocket expenses are becoming more common.

Summary

One of the most widely used health indexes is the age-adjusted mortality rate. Most of the industrialized countries of the world have lower age-specific death rates than occur in the United States in spite of the much greater per capita expenditures on health in the latter. This finding raises important questions regarding the efficiency and effectiveness of the United States' health system.

The health services industry is characterized by a number of particular characteristics that distinguish it from those industries more directly affected by market forces. These features include consumer ignorance, the nonprofit aspect of much of the industry, and the restrictions on competition that are implemented by various associations of health providers.

Expenditures for medical services have risen rapidly since World War II and now amount to 7.7 percent of gross national product. While much of the increase in expenditures is due to increased utilization, a large part is accounted for by a rapid and sustained medical price inflation. The latter, which is most closely associated with wage increases, advances in technology, and the marked rise in the demand for health services, has been most severe with respect to hospitals.

Since 1940 the health insurance industry has grown rapidly. However, because of gaps in benefit coverage, as well as the inability of the insurance industry to provide coverage for the very poor, there has been an increase in legislative proposals for a more active public role in the provision of health insurance.

Notes

1. Victor R. Fuchs, *Essays in the Economics of Health and Medical Care* (New York: National Bureau of Economic Research, 1972), pp. 3-4.

2. Fuchs, *Essays*, p. 10.

3. R.H. Johnson, "The Health of Israel," *The Lancet*, 7417, October 23, 1965, p. 845.

4. B.S. Sanders, "Measuring Community Health Levels," *American Journal of Public Health*, Vol. 54, July 1964, pp. 1063-70.

5. National Center for Health Statistics: An Index of Health, Mathematical Models, by C.L. Chiang, *Vital and Health Statistics.* PHS Publication No. 1000-Series 2-No. 5, Public Health Service (Washington, D.C.: U.S. Government Printing Office, May 1965).

6. Daniel F. Sullivan, *Conceptual Problems in Developing an Index of Health*, Health Resources Publication 74-1017 (Washington, D.C.: U.S. Government Printing Office, 1974), p. 4.

7. Karen Davis has argued that, in fact, nonprofit hospitals do make substantial profits. See Karen Davis, "Economic Theories of Behavior in Nonprofit Private Hospitals," *Economic and Business Bulletin*, Vol. 24, No. 2, August 1972, p. 8.

8. Alan Gregg, *Challenges to Contemporary Medicine* (New York: Columbia University Press, 1956).

9. Herbert E. Klarman, *The Economics of Health* (New York: Columbia University Press, 1965), p. 12. Events that happen to individuals on a fairly regular basis cannot be insured because the premiums would exceed the cost of the event occurring. Events that are unpredictable and occur only occasionally to individuals can be insured because many individuals pay insurance premiums but experience no reimbursable expense. Therefore premiums for all are lower than the cost associated with the event occurring.

10. Alfred M. Skolnik and Sophie R. Dales, "Social Welfare Expenditures, 1972-1973," *Social Security Bulletin*, Vol. 37, No. 1, January 1974, p. 13.

18

11. Herman M. Somers, "Economic Issues in Health Services," in Neil W. Chamberlain, *Contemporary Economic Issues* (Homewood, Illinois: Richard D. Irwin, 1969), p. 110.

12. Skolnik and Dales, "Social Welfare Expenditures," p. 14.

13. U.S. Bureau of the Census, 1970 Census of Population, *Industrial Characteristics*, Subject Reports, PC(2)-7B (Washington, D.C.: U.S. Government Printing Office, 1973), p. 4.

14. U.S. Department of Health, Education, and Welfare, National Center for Health Statistics, *Health Manpower, U.S. 1965-1967* (Series 14, No. 1), (Washington, D.C.: U.S. Government Printing Office, 1968), p. 53.

15. Barbara S. Cooper, Nancy L. Worthington, and Paula A. Piro, "National Health Expenditures, 1929-1973," *Social Security Bulletin*, Vol. 37, No. 2, February 1974, pp. 8-10.

16. Somers, "Economic Issues," p. 111.

17. Herbert E. Klarman, Dorothy P. Rice, Barbara S. Cooper, and H. Louis Stettler, III, *Source of Increase in Selected Medical Care Expenditures*, Social Security Administration, Office of Research and Statistics, Staff Paper No. 4 (Washington, D.C.: U.S. Government Printing Office, 1970), p. 4.

18. Klarman, et al., *Increase in Selected Medical Care Expenditures*, p. 39.

19. Cooper, et al., "National Health Expenditures," pp. 75-76.

20. Anne A. Scitovsky, "Changes in the Cost of Treatment of Selected Illnesses, 1951-1965," *American Economic Review*, Vol. 57, December 1967, pp. 1182-95.

21. Harold Goldstein, "Health and Medical Care," in Gustav Schuckster and Edwin Dale, Jr., *The Economist Looks at Society* (Lexington, Massachusetts: Xerox Publishing Co., 1973), p. 169.

22. Ibid. The minimum utilization rate required to justify purchase of such equipment will vary somewhat from item to item.

23. U.S. Department of Health, Education and Welfare, *Medical Care Costs and Prices, 1972* (Washington, D.C.: U.S. Government Printing Office, 1972), p. 112.

24. *The Baltimore Evening Sun*, October 4, 1974, p. B-3.

25. Milton I. Roemer, "On Paying the Doctor and the Implications of Different Methods," in Roy H. Elling (Ed.), *National Health Care: Issues and Problems in Socialized Medicine* (New York: Aldine-Atherton, Inc., 1971), p. 127.

26. Roemer, "On Paying the Doctor," p. 132.

27. HEW, *Medical Care Costs and Prices*, p. 97. Although insurance coverage varies greatly by income levels this should not be construed to mean that a large proportion of the poor are unable to obtain medical care.

28. In addition to its effect on costs, restrictive health insurance likely has deleterious effects on the quality of care. See, for example, A.P. Ingegno, "Bad Insurance Means Bad Medical Practice," *Medical Economics*, April 29, 1968, pp. 171-83.

29. Somers, "Economic Issues," p. 119.

2 The Demand for Health Services

What does the economist mean by the concept of demand? *Demand* for a good is defined as the various quantities of a commodity that consumers will purchase at all possible alternative prices, other things equal. The quantity that consumers will buy is affected by a number of factors, including: (1) price of the good; (2) consumers' tastes and preferences: (3) consumers' incomes; and (4) prices of related goods.[1]

Demand refers to an entire schedule or demand curve. A *demand schedule* indicates the various quantities of the commodity that consumers will purchase given alternative prices of the commodity. A hypothetical demand schedule is shown in Table 2-1.

A *demand curve* is a demand schedule plotted on an ordinary graph. A demand curve is shown in Figure 2-1. The vertical axis of the graph measures price per unit. The horizontal axis measures quantity of the commodity purchased per unit of time. Note that the inverse relationship between price and quantity sold makes the demand curve slope downward to the right.

The demand curve represents the *maximum* quantities that consumers will purchase at various prices. At given prices they would always be willing to purchase smaller amounts (if lesser amounts were all they could obtain), but they will not purchase more than the amount shown by the demand curve. The demand curve can also be viewed as indicating the maximum prices that consumers will pay for different quantities per unit of time. They are not willing to pay more but will certainly pay less for each of the various quantities.[2]

A clear distinction must be made between movement along a given demand curve and a shift in the curve itself. The former is termed an increase or decrease in the *quantity demanded*, while the latter is known as a *change in demand*. A change in the quantity demanded results from variations in the price of the good, with all other factors affecting the quantity purchased remaining unchanged. For example, in Figure 2-2 a decrease in price from P to P_1 increases the quantity demanded from X to X_1. When the factors held constant in defining a given state of demand change, the demand curve itself will change. Thus, in Figure 2-2 an increase in consumers' incomes will shift the demand curve to the right from DD to D_1D_1. A shift in consumer preferences to commodity X and away from other goods will have the same result.

Elasticity

Price elasticity refers to the responsiveness of the quantity demanded to changes in the price of the product, all other factors being held constant. Alfred Marshall

19

Table 2-1
Price and Quantities Demanded (Per Unit of Time)

Price	Quantity (Per Unit Time)
24	0
22	3
20	6
18	9
16	12
14	15
12	18
10	21
8	24
6	27

first developed the coefficient of elasticity, which is defined as the percentage change in quantity demanded divided by the percentage change in price, when the price change is small.[3] In terms of algebra, the elasticity definition appears as:

$$\epsilon = \frac{\dfrac{\Delta X}{X}}{\dfrac{-\Delta P}{P}}$$

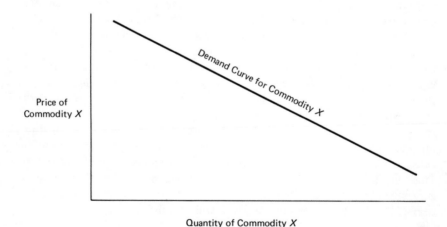

Figure 2-1. Demand Curve for Commodity X

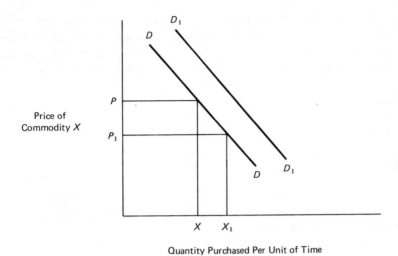

Figure 2-2. Change in Demand for Commodity X

The formula can be visualized by reference to Figure 2-2. The mathematical symbol Δ means "small change in." The change in quantity from X to X_1 is ΔX. The change in price from P to P_1 is ΔP. The number or coefficient denoting elasticity is obtained by dividing a percentage by a percentage and is a pure number independent of any unit of measurement. When the elasticity coefficient is less than one, demand is defined to be inelastic; when the coefficient is greater than one, demand is elastic; and when the coefficient is equal to one, demand is considered to be of unitary elasticity. There are three important factors that influence elasticity of demand for a commodity. These are (1) the availability of substitutes for the commodity; (2) the number of alternative uses for the commodity; and (3) the price of the commodity relative to consumers' incomes.

The availability of substitutes is probably the most important factor enumerated. If close substitutes are readily available, demand for a given commodity will tend to be elastic. For example, if the price of margarine falls while the price of butter remains unchanged, consumers will tend to purchase more margarine and less butter.

The greater the number of uses for a given commodity, the more elastic will be the demand for it. Suppose that steel could only be used in the making of automobiles. There would be little likelihood for much variation in quantity purchased as its price changed, and demand for steel would be inelastic. However, steel can in fact be used in the manufacture of hundreds of items. The possible variation in quantity purchased is quite large and tends to make the demand for steel more elastic.

Demand for commodities that account for a large fraction of the consumer's income will be more elastic than those that are only a small proportion of total consumer expenditures. Thus, goods such as air conditioners, which require large outlays, make consumers price-conscious. Quantity demanded is likely to vary considerably in response to price changes. For items such as salt, which account for a negligible fraction of consumer incomes, changes in price are likely to have little effect on the quantity demanded.

The Engel Curve

A demand curve indicates the different quantities of one good that the consumer will purchase at various possible *prices*, other things being equal. An *Engel curve* shows the different quantities of one good that the consumer will purchase at various levels of *income*, other things being equal.[4] Engel curves for two different types of commodities are shown in Figure 2-3.

Engel curves provide useful information regarding consumption patterns for various commodities and for different individuals. For basic items such as food, as the consumer's income increases from very low levels, his consumption may increase considerably. However, as his income continues to rise, the increases in consumption become less than proportional to the income gains. This is illustrated in Figure 2-3A. For other items such as recreation or luxury goods, expenditures tend to increase in greater proportion than income. The Engel curve presented in Figure 2-3B reflects this situation.

Income elasticity refers to the responsiveness of the quantity purchased to changes in income. When the percentage change in the quantity purchased is

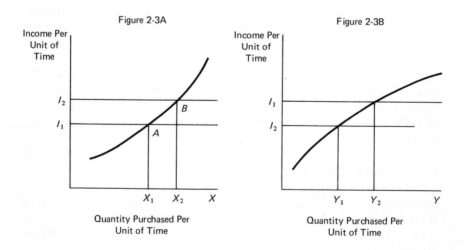

Figure 2-3. Engel Curves

smaller than the percentage change in income, the commodity has an income elasticity coefficient that is less than one. However, should the percentage change in the quantity purchased be greater than the percentage change in income, then the income elasticity coefficient would be greater than one. If the percentage change in the quantity purchased is equal to the percentage change in income, the income elasticity coefficient is equal to one.

The Demand for Health Services

As indicated in the previous chapter, most observers agree that consumers are more ignorant and uncertain in their role as consumers of health services than as purchasers of most other commodities. They cannot assess the quality and character of the health services they consume and are generally unaware of the variety of health care alternatives available for treating a given illness.[5] Ethical standards adopted by the health professions preclude advertising, so consumers are denied access to this form of information concerning the relative merits and costs of various forms of care and treatment. Moreover, the reluctance of some physicians to discuss illness in nontechnical terms also tends to keep consumers ignorant of feasible treatment alternatives and makes it nearly impossible for them to exercise rational choice. While individuals may choose their physicians, doctors usually determine the kind and quantity of health services individuals consume. While doctors may have some knowledge of the individual's financial resources, there is little evidence that these considerations have much influence on the type of care prescribed.

Consumers also generally lack knowledge concerning their actual need for care. Except for some obvious conditions such as pain, bleeding, or impaired abilities, individuals frequently do not recognize symptoms of illness or realize the consequences of failing to obtain prompt treatment. While the incidence of illness can be predicted with reasonable accuracy for groups of health consumers, sickness for an individual is often unpredictable. Moreover, the speed of recovery from illness is often difficult to forecast. Thus, the overall benefit of health services is generally uncertain from the consumer's point of view, and the demand for a sizable fraction of health services is based on the doctor's judgment.

This should not imply, however, that the consumer completely relinquishes control over the consumption decision to the physician. He always has the option of not following the physician's advice. A more important choice mechanism, however, is through one's selection of physician. Many patients are known to change physicians until they find one who will provide the type of treatment they want. A more subtle method is through choice of a regular physician who reflects the desires of one's socioeconomic group.[6]

In the areas of public health, medical education, and medical research, demand is exercised collectively through nonprofit organizations and government rather than individually. It is only when the family looks after its own health needs without benefit of professional advice and the services of health care institutions, that individual consumer choice can be said to be freely operable. An example is the area of nonprescription drugs. The effects of the partial insulation of consumer demand from free market forces are not fully known; but it is likely that the behavior of demand (for example, the responses to changed prices) is quite different than in a market of "direct consumer sovereignty."[7]

As indicated previously, the demand and need for medical care is not always the same. For instance, an individual may demand more care than is required medically. Conversely, he may need medical care but may not be aware of its value. Moreover, specialized facilities and services could be unavailable to him or he could be without funds to purchase sufficient medical services. Need is generated by the incidence of illness, while demand is generated by the interrelationship of illness with other factors. To plan for future use of facilities and personnel, demand rather than need for such resources must be projected.

To the extent that expenditures on medical care primarily reflect a "need" rather than a "want," economic variables will show little or no relation to expenditures on medical care; that is, income and price differences will have little or no effect on expenditures if the effect of need is overwhelming. However, if there is a significant relationship between medical care expenditures and several economic variables (in addition to variables that represent health status), then demand theory is of significant value in explaining family expenditures for medical care.[8]

There is some basis for assuming that demand analysis can be applied with appropriate modifications to explain variations in expenditures on medical care services. From the patient's viewpoint, the need for medical care is not always clear-cut. For example, the distinction between a severe cold and pneumonia may not be noticeable to the consumer. Chest pains may indicate either bronchitis or a serious heart condition. In such instances a high-income family would be expected to take greater precautions and thus incur higher medical care expenditures than a low-income family. Moreover, even after treatment is begun, economic factors may influence its duration. A poor family may decide to forego the possible benefit from an extra day in the hospital or an additional visit to the physician.

Medical care is characterized by a low degree of substitutability. Most medical needs are highly specific and alternative goods are not able to supply the same level of satisfaction. Moreover, medical care is generally not wanted for its own sake. Most medical care and treatment is unpleasant, and generally is not wanted until it becomes a preferable alternative to the pain and other consequences of illness. This implies that the price elasticity of demand for medical care would tend to be low.

Grover C. Wirick has identified five fundamental factors that can have an impact on the demand for health care services.[9] The first is need. A person suffers from a condition that requires attention, or he has some other reason for seeking medical care or examination.

Second, there must be a realization of need. Either the individual or someone acting in his behalf must know that the need exists. A number of psychological processes probably are involved including awareness of the existence and availability of medical skills as well as the benefit likely to be gained through health services. Intertwined with these elements are the hopes, fears, and beliefs of the individual, as well as other personal factors such as his previous experiences, customs, and religion.[10] For example, a person with a strong religious conviction against a particular kind of medical treatment may have a different realization of the need for care from that of someone with other religious beliefs.

Third, financial resources must be available to implement the care. This capability may take many forms, including the income and assets possessed by the individual or his family, insurance coverage, eligibility for free care under a group or government program, and availability of care through welfare programs. An individual's financial resources for medical care may be different from those for other items in his budget and may even differ from one kind of medical care to another. Thus, many health insurance policies may give one almost complete accessibility to hospital care but may leave dental care unavailable.

Fourth, there must be a specific motivation to obtain the needed care. Even with the other forces present—need, realization, and resources—something must initiate the action. Going to the doctor with an acute condition involving pain or bleeding is caused by the condition itself, but the motivation is less clear with respect to other types of medical care. This force is also related to willingness to obtain care, but it is more inclusive. Rather than being only a static readiness to accept medical help, this factor implies an active move toward obtaining it.[11] For example, a physician can recommend hospitalization, but the patient must have himself admitted. A more general example, based on cultural predispositions, is the idea that an individual should go to the dentist at least once a year.

Fifth is availability of service. The first three forces are characteristics of the patient, while the fifth is a phenomenon of his environment. The fourth force is somewhat indistinct and could be characteristic of either or both.

Difficulties in Estimating the Demand for Medical Care

As implied above, economists usually describe the demand for a good or service as being determined by its own price, the prices of other goods and services, consumer income, and consumer tastes.

Most providers of health care are price setters rather than price takers. Therefore, prices may remain constant for long periods while variations in demand result in changes in rates of utilization rather than increases or decreases in price. This type of seller behavior greatly increases the difficulty of estimating price elasticities of demand.[12] Conceptually, in order to estimate demand curves for a typical individual one would need a set of data on individuals with very similar characteristics who are charged different prices. The existence of third party or insurance payments for some, but not all individuals, or the existence of differing proportions of insurance coverage can help to generate such information.

Moreover, survey data of consumer expenditures on health services cannot be expected to be of any help in estimating price elasticities of demand since price information is not included in such data. In contrast, patient discharge statistics that contained information regarding different proportions of third party payments among patients might be useful for estimating price elasticities of demand. However, this latter information would not contain data on the prices of substitute goods or services that were not consumed. Thus, we would not expect prices of substitutes to be included in empirical estimates of the demand for health care. Lacking information on substitutes for medical care services makes it impossible to measure cross elasticities of demand.[a]

What is the appropriate dependent variable in medical care demand studies? One writer has suggested that it is the dollar amount a person spends, since for a given expenditure the physician will provide a certain treatment.[13] However, an empirical measure such as medical care expenditures may bias the effects of the factors believed to influence demand (prices and income), if it is not first adjusted for price changes and for variations in the quality of the product itself. These problems are present in both time-series and cross-section analysis.[b] For example, per capita medical care expenditures are a combination of both the price charged for the treatment and the number of treatments obtained. If a rise in patient's economic resources is accompanied by a rise in medical care expenditures, the latter may be merely the result of either an increase in the price to the patient (the sliding scale fee schedule) or an increase in his consumption of medical care services per se.[c]

---

[a]Cross elasticity of demand measures the extent to which various commodities are economically related to each other. If we consider commodities X and Y, the cross elasticity of X with respect to Y equals the percentage change in the quantity of X purchased divided by the percentage change in the price of Y. This can be expressed mathematically by

$$\theta XY = \frac{\Delta X/X}{\Delta P_Y/P_Y}$$

[b]Nearly all studies of the demand for medical care are cross-sectional. A time-series study reflects the influence of a multitude of factors that cannot be separated. However, by examining data for a cross section of families in the same time period, the effect of factors influencing their health expenditures can be assessed while holding constant the state of technology and other conditions with change over time.

[c]Before health insurance became widespread, the practice of using sliding scale fees was commonplace. (A form of price discrimination.) However, this practice has apparently declined greatly with the expansion of third-party payments.

Physical measures such as doctor visits or length of stay in the hospital also have their disadvantages. Not only are these variables heterogeneous (especially with respect to quality), but these measures also fail to reflect changes in the state of the art and in medical technology.

The effect of income on the demand for health care cannot be predicted with certainty a priori. An estimated income elasticity of expenditure greater than unity might imply that the proportion of income spent for health care would rise as income rises, while an elasticity of less than unity might imply that a declining proportion of income would be spent for health care as income increases. However, the effect of medical research, which may discover new means of treating diseases, new surgical procedures, and new drugs, may be to provide new goods and services for the consumer, thereby increasing health care expenditures over that which would be predicted by the estimated income elasticities of expenditures.[14]

Moreover, the demand for health care may depend on expected future income as well as on current income. Therefore an estimate of the average of current and future incomes, which is called "permanent income," is sometimes used in demand studies instead of current income.[15] This is because measured income is an imperfect indicator of "normal" or "permanent" income since it consists of both permanent and transitory components. These two components are assumed to be uncorrelated. One test of the permanent income hypothesis is to see whether the income elasticity of demand is associated less closely with measured than permanent income.[16]

Consumption patterns of individuals may affect their general health and thereby their demand for health care. Individuals with higher incomes may have had better nutrition and better health care in the past and these factors may lower their current demand for health care. However, this would be offset by their ability to buy more health care because of their higher incomes. If individuals with higher incomes are in better health, then this would tend to lower the estimated income elasticity of expenditures.

Studies have shown that more educated populations tend to have better health than less educated ones even at the same levels of income, expenditures for medical care, and other variables.[17] However, researchers have disagreed on whether education increases or decreases demand.

To the extent that education induces behavior that is designed to increase satisfaction in the future, one might expect that education would increase the demand for medical care, all other things being equal. This would be most likely to be true for those kinds of care with a large investment component, and particularly for ambulatory rather than inpatient services.[18] However, greater prevention and treatment earlier in the course of illness could reduce the total amount of medical care ultimately demanded through positive effects on overall health status. Differences between studies of the estimated effect of education on demand may stem from differences in the health status of individuals included in each body of data.

As implied above, the primary determinant of an individual's demand for health care is his actual health status. For example, an individual's partial deafness may generate a demand for a hearing aid. His financial status and the prices of hearing aids would then affect the amount he would spend on them. However, a person with normal hearing would not purchase a hearing aid no matter what the prices of hearing aids or his income might be.

Some of the determinants of an individual's physical condition are his health habits, such as cigarette smoking, age, and urban or rural residence. However, one of the unsolved problems in the analysis of demand for health services is the construction of an adequate health index that would be used as an independent variable in a demand equation.

Empirical Research

Empirical studies of demand have two purposes: The first is explanation—the ability to specify and estimate the relationship between use of a product or service and the factors influencing its use. The other important application of this kind of study is prediction of future demand. Such estimates can serve, for example, as guides for determining the numbers and types of health personnel or medical care facilities required in the future.

Grover C. Wirick and Robin Barlow examined the determinants of the medical expenditures of a sample of Michigan families during 1957-58.[19] The statistical technique that was utilized was analysis of variance which is equivalent to multiple regression when all of the independent variables are dummy variables.

The dependent variable was the sum of individual expenditures for medical care (including amounts contributed by sources outside the family but excluding health insurance premiums). The independent (dummy) variables were limited to the following seven categories: (1) age of individual; (2) insurance coverage; (3) family income; (4) number of equivalent adults; (5) responses to minor symptoms; (6) education of family head; and (7) residence of family head as a youth.

The analysis was carried out separately for each sex. (See Table 2-2.)

For both males and females, the independent variables only explained about 8 percent of the variation in medical care expenditures. The age-class variables accounted for about one-half of the explained variation for males and about three-quarters of the explained variation for females. Medical expenditures were thus shown to be positively related to the age of the individual.

The authors concluded that "consumption seems to be determined in large part by needs which are more or less randomly distributed in the population, but also tends to be restricted by limited resources. This indicates that medical expenditures are highly regressive. . . ."[20]

Paul J. Feldstein utilized data obtained in a 1958 survey of American families to estimate a series of demand curves for health care. The primary results are summarized in Table 2-3. Because the equations are presented in double logarithmic form the coefficients indicate the elasticity of the various independent variables with respect to the appropriate dependent variable. Asterisks indicate that the independent variable is significant at the 5 percent level.

As indicated in Table 2-3 the mean family income variable was significant in three of the five equations. The indicated income elasticity (Engel curve) of 0.5 or 0.6 is somewhat lower than that found by George J. Stigler[21] in an earlier study, but approximately the same as the income elasticity calculated by the author utilizing data from a 1970 survey of health expenditure.[22]

Health insurance coverage was positively related to total medical care expenditures, hospital patient days, and hospital expenditures. In each case this relationship was statistically significant. This is consistent with the findings of the Wirick-Barlow study, which also indicated that people with health insurance coverage tend to have higher out-of-pocket medical costs. There are a number of possible explanations for this phenomenon. One possibility is that the insured are charged higher fees, so that the value of their insurance benefit is partly vitiated. A second factor is that insurance tends to lead to the abuse of benefits. Consistent with this possibility is the fact that persons with two or more insurance policies have a higher hospital admission rate than those with a single policy. Moreover, the adverse selection of risks may be a factor, too; that is, persons in poor health may be more inclined to secure multiple coverage than persons in good health.[23]

In addition, because insurance coverage causes the price of certain health services provided a patient to be relatively low, a larger quantity of services may be obtained than in the absence of insurance. Thus, some out-of-pocket expenditures would usually be required. Finally, the insured may have both superior appreciation of and ability to pay for health and medical care.

Paul J. Feldstein developed two price variables. The physician price variable was obtained by dividing net expenditures on physicians by doctor visits. The hospital care price variable was obtained by dividing net expenditures on hospital care by the quantity of hospital care. The coefficient of the price variable had the expected negative sign (−0.19) only when physician visits was the dependent variable.[d] (See Table 2-3.) When the dependent variable was one of the expenditure items, the coefficient of the price variable was positive. Since expenditure consists of price times quantity, price and expenditure would tend to be positively correlated.[24]

Victor Fuchs found, as did Feldstein, that the price elasticity of demand for physicians' services is low (−0.36).[25] Why is medical care demand relatively insensitive to price? One reason is that the demand for physicians' services is derived from the consumer's demand for health. Michael Grossman has esti-

---

[d]Because traditional demand theory indicates that price and quantity demanded are inversely related, one would expect the sign of the coefficient to be negative.

Table 2-2
A Multivariate Analysis Explaining Variations in the Medical Expenditures of Michigan Individuals, 1957-58

Individual Characteristic	MALE Grand Mean = $74		FEMALE Grand Mean = $103	
	Deviation of Class Mean from Grand Mean	Percent of Variance Explained	Deviation Class Mean from Grand Mean	Percent of Variance Explained
Age of Individual		4.0		6.0
	$		$	
Under 5	−26		−58	
5-14	−22		−53	
15-44	− 6		27	
45-64	42		23	
65-69	84		37	
70 and over	42		63	
Insurance Coverage		1.0		1.2
None	−17		−33	
Poorly insured	−10		13	
Moderately insured	6		6	
Highly insured	22		20	
Family Income		0.7		0.7
Under 2,000	22		21	
2,000-4,000	− 6		0	
4,000-6,000	−12		− 7	

	(1)	(2)
6,000-7,500	4	2
7,500-10,000	4	-15
10,000 and over	22	34
Number of Adults	1.0	0.4
1.0	2	3
1.5-2.0	19	10
2.5-4.0	-3	-1
4.5 and over	-11	-10
Response to Minor Symptoms	0.3	0.3
Would visit doctor promptly	11	10
Depends	-1	-4
Would wait	-12	-12
Do not know	-16	3
Education of Head	0.5	0.1
Under 9 years	6	-5
9-12	-6	0
College	8	8
Where Head Grew Up	0.2	0.2
Urban U.S. except South	3	2
Rural U.S. except South	1	-6
South-urban	-17	-6
South-rural	-11	-6
Non-U.S.	3	17

Source: Grover Wirick and Robin Barlow, "The Economic and Social Determinants of the Demand for Health Services," in *The Economics of Health and Medical Care*, Bureau of Public Health Economics (Ann Arbor, Michigan: University of Michigan, 1964), p. 117.

Table 2-3
Summary of Logarithmic Regression Results

Dependent Variable	Mean Family Income	Age of Head	% Families One or More Members Over 65	% Families One or More Members Under 5 Years	% Urban	% Families Receiving Free or Reduced Care	% Families 12 or More Years of Education	Mean Family Size	Family Type	Insurance	Price Variable	R^2
Gross medical care expenditures	0.59*	0.24	−0.05	+0.06	−0.01	0.02	−0.18*	−0.17	−0.03	+0.09*	——	0.33
Physician visits	.62*	.10	.05	.08	−.01	.04	−.25*	−.07	−.10	−.01	−0.19*	.33
Physician expenditures	.56*	−0.41	.04	.02	.00	.00	−.11	−.13	−.10	.10	.02	.28
Hospital patient days	.47	3.48*	−.04	.46*	.06	−.10	−.24	1.17*	.02	.25*	.01	.32
Hospital expenditures	0.50	1.60	−0.13	0.19	0.03	−0.10	−0.28*	0.49	0.02	0.48*	0.43*	0.55

*Significant at the 5 percent level

Source: American Medical Association, *Report of the Commission on the Cost of Medical Care*, Vol. 1, General Report (Chicago, Illinois: American Medical Association, 1964), p. 74.

mated the price elasticity of demand for health at −0.5, which seems reasonable given the absence of any close substitutes for health.[26] The price elasticity of demand for a derived input (physicians' services) must be lower than for the final commodity (health) unless there are major substitution possibilities with other inputs. Moreover, there are many legal and psychological barriers against the substitution of persons without the M.D. degree in the physicians' role, even though such persons might be good substitutes in a technical sense.

Ronald Anderson and Lee Benham tested the hypothesis that there was a greater income elasticity of demand for physician and dental services if the independent variable was permanent income rather than current income. After controlling for differences in the price and quality of care as well as a number of demographic variables, they found that the permanent income elasticity of demand for physicians' services was *lower* than the current income elasticity; for dental services the opposite result occurred. Anderson and Benham explain this unexpected finding regarding physician services by stating that, "The secular increase in the consumption of hospital and physician services would appear to be less closely related to income per se and more closely related to other factors such as the changing methods of financing medical care."[27]

If hospital usage were determined solely by medical factors, then the price elasticity of demand for hospital services would be zero. However, economic factors may introduce some elasticity into the demand function. The importance of economic factors may differ among illnesses and conditions.

Gerald Rosenthal examined the effect of two alternative "price variables" (average daily room charge and cash outlay as a percentage of the total bill) on the length of stay of hospital patients. The data consisted of a sample of medical records and financial information from the year 1962 for patients who were in 68 New England hospitals.

Rosenthal divided the data into 28 groups, which were homogeneous with respect to medical or surgical diagnosis, age, and sex. For each of the 28 groups, he related length of stay to the two independent price variables.

Since Rosenthal utilized double-log regressions, the coefficient of the independent variable is an estimate of the elasticity of the dependent variable with respect to the independent variable. However, neither of the two independent variables is own price. Therefore, the elasticities that are indicated below are not price elasticities of demand.

For most of the medical categories the elasticity of cash/total bill with respect to length of stay is 0.02 or less; the elasticity of average daily room charge with respect to length of stay varied generally from 0.2 to 0.4.[28] Moreover, for over half the categories, the elasticity with respect to the latter independent variable was significant at the 5 percent level, while the elasticity when considering the former independent variable was almost never significant.

The analysis could be summarized as some evidence of significant price elasticity when the price variable is the average daily room charge. This particular price variable is most likely to be known by the patient, since it conforms quite closely to the stated daily room charge posted by the institution. It is interesting that much less price elasticity of demand is demonstrated with respect to relative cash outlay, although the actual cash outlay would be expected to influence the utilization of the facility by the patient. It is likely that the actual cash outlay and the cash outlay relative to the total bill is not known by the patient until the moment of discharge from the institution and is therefore not likely to motivate him to reduce the length of his stay. On the other hand, the $90 to $100 daily room charge is better known to the patient and is likely to be quite influential in determining his behavior.[29]

Fuchs has criticized Rosenthal's study on a number of grounds. He points out that an investigation of price elasticity should have quantity as the dependent variable and price and other relevant factors as independent variables. However, in Rosenthal's paper, the dependent variable is length of stay, not the quantity of hospital services. Since length of stay is correlated with the admission rate and the number of services per day, the elasticities are presumably biased estimates of the true quantity-price elasticities.[30] Moreover, the price variable, average daily room charge, is calculated by dividing the total room charge by length of stay. The appearance of the dependent variable as a denominator in the independent variable does introduce the possibility of some negative regression bias.[31]

Hyman Joseph related third-party payments to length of stay in Iowa hospitals for 22 separate illnesses or conditions. The estimates of the coefficient of the third party payments variable were statistically significant in seven of the 22 diagnostic categories.[32] Third-party payments appeared to have little effect on length of stay for illnesses or conditions that require extensive care or are psychologically unpleasant. However, third-party payments did appear to effect length of stay for the less-serious illnesses or conditions.

The price elasticities of demand that were computed for a representative patient were generally low. Elastic demands (price elasticity >1) were computed only for two categories in which outpatient care might be a reasonable substitute for an extra day in the hospital. These were primary atypical pneumonia and fracture of neck femur. Joseph's analysis also indicated that patients with higher priced accommodations tended to have longer stays.[33] These results are consistent with a positive income effect.

Recent research has focused on the demand for health insurance. Fuchs and Marcia Kramer, using cross-section data from 1966, investigated the demand for physician office care insurance using interstate aggregated data. The dependent variable is the absolute level of benefits (BEN). They found BEN to be highly related to income (elasticities ranged from 0.76 to 1.61) and also highly own-price sensitive, with elasticities varying from -1.58 to -1.74.[34] They also found that benefits were strongly negatively related to medical prices. Charles E. Phelps found an own-price elasticity for physician visit coverage, using 1963 data of -0.5,[35] which is considerably below that found by Fuchs and Kramer but much higher than estimates of the price elasticity of demand for physician office care itself.[e] (See Table 2-3.)

This type of research has important policy implications because of the possible introduction of national health insurance. For example, if the purchase of supplementary insurance is highly sensitive to medical care prices (which the Fuchs–Kramer results imply), then large demand shifts within the medical care system via comprehensive national health insurance could be exacerbated through purchase of supplemental insurance policies.

The Demand for Dental Services

Because the demand for dental care is more closely related to economic determinants than need, the income elasticity of demand for dental care is higher than for physicians services. (See Table 2-4.)

The type of dental treatment demanded varies according to family income.

Table 2-4
Income Elasticities of Physicians' and Dentists' Services, Selected Studies

Study	Income Elasticity of Physicians' Services	Income Elasticity of Dental Services
Anderson-Benham (1970)	0.22	0.61
Rosenthal (1964)	0.56	1.17
Feldstein and Carr (1964)	0.50	--
Stigler (1952)	0.52-0.81	--
Newhouse (1970)	0.7-0.9	1.6
Upton-Silverman (1972)	--	2.3
Feldstein (1972)	--	1.7

Source: Ronald Anderson and Lee Benham, "Factors Affecting the Relationship Between Family Income and Medical Care Consumption," in Herbert E. Klarman (Ed.), *Empirical Studies in Health Economics* (Baltimore, Maryland: Johns Hopkins Press, © 1970), p. 86; Gerald Rosenthal, "The Demand for Medical Care," in *Report of the Commission on the Cost of Medical Care* (Chicago, Illinois: American Medical Association, 1964), p. 74; Paul Felstein and John Carr, "The Effect of Income on Medical Care Spending," *Proceedings of the Social Statistics Section of the American Statistical Association*, Vol. 7, 1964; George J. Stigler, *The Theory of Price* (New York: Macmillan, 1952); Charles Upton and William Silverman, "The Demand for Dental Services," *Journal of Human Resources*, Vol. 7, No. 2, Spring 1972, p. 253; Paul J. Feldstein, *Financing Dental Care: An Economic Analysis* (Cambridge, Massachusetts: Heath Lexington, 1973), p. 39; and Joseph Newhouse, "A Model of Physician Pricing," *The Southern Economic Journal*, Vol. 37, No. 1, October 1970, p. 180.

[e]Fuchs and Kramer found that the elasticities of demand with respect to income, price, and insurance were all small relative to the direct effect of the number of physicians on demand. Because physicians are able to affect the demand for their services to a considerable extent, one should be skeptical of proposals which argue that the cost of medical care would be decreased by augmenting the supply of physicians.

Lower income families will have a greater proportionate demand for dentures and extractions than will higher income families. Those with higher incomes are likely to demand more preventive and maintenance work such as fillings, examinations, cleanings, straightenings, and gum treatment.[36]

Charles Upton and William Silverman have estimated the effects of flourida-tion on the future demand for dental services.[37] They assume that real incomes will double over the next 40 years and if the full effects of flouridation are experienced, the per capita demand for selected services should change by the proportions given in the first column of Table 2-5.

The estimates given in column one do not allow for any response to a change in the price of dentists' services. However, in the long run the price (wage) of dentists must be equal to wage rates in occupations requiring similar levels of skill and education. In the absence of what the authors believed were reasonable estimates of the price elasticity of demand for dentists' services, they arbitrarily assumed that it is equal to −1. Given the additional assumption of a doubling in the price of dental services the adjusted per capita demand for selected services is indicated in the second column of Table 2-5.

Thus, to the extent that the assumptions indicated above are correct, the number of dentists per capita would remain relatively constant over the next generation; work would be directed less to simple restorations and extractions and more to complicated services such as dentures.

Suggestions for Further Research

As indicated previously, economists have generally failed to include measures of health status as independent variables in demand analyses. If health status is as important as it appears, its effect on demand for health services should be studied rather than avoided.[38] Economists frequently indicate that little is

Table 2-5
Forecasts of Per Capita Demand for Dental Services in 40 Years

Service	No Price Adjustment	Price Adjustment
Restorations	−56%	−78%
Prophylaxis	60	−20
Extractions	−72	−86
Bridges and dentures	243	72
Dentists	105	2

Source: Charles Upton and William Silverman, "The Demand for Dental Services," *Journal of Human Resources*, Vol. 7, No. 2 (© 1972 by the Regents of the University of Wisconsin), p. 261.

known about the effectiveness of medical services in improving health. However, instead of attempting to augment the limited knowledge in this area, they often put their efforts into demand studies that omit health.

When health is omitted from a demand analysis, its effects become subsumed under those of income and other variables with which it is correlated. The inclusion of a separate health variable would make it possible to estimate the effects of changes in health on medical care demand and to obtain better estimates of the effects of other variables. The effects of omission of health on other variables can easily be illustrated. Consider a range of incomes in which improvements in earnings are associated with gains in health. A regression analysis omitting health status would tend to underestimate the income elasticities of demand. Moreover, it is known that hospitalization rates vary little by income-size class, but physicians' office visits per capita vary considerably. This may be because the latter reduce the demand for hospital services by virtue of their impact on health.

A second area in which research is needed is the role played by time in determining the demand for medical care. As out-of-pocket costs are reduced because of either the spread of private insurance or the enactment of a federal health insurance program, demand will become more responsive to time prices. This will permit persons with a lower opportunity cost of time to bid services away from those with a higher opportunity cost because the former face a lower price. In a study of outpatient visits to New York City Municipal Hospitals, Jan Paul Acton found that the elasticity of demand with respect to distance was −2.07 suggesting that the time price elasticity of demand is considerably greater than the own price elasticity of demand.[39]

Summary

The first portion of the chapter develops part of the elementary theory of consumer demand. The nature of the demand curve as well as the concepts of price and income elasticity are defined and explained, and some factors affecting the elasticity of demand are discussed.

A number of difficulties, both of a conceptual and empirical nature, which arise in estimating the demand for health services, were enumerated. These include a lack of information concerning medical care prices, the problems which arise in developing an adequate dependent variable in medical care demand studies, and the nonexistence of an overall health index to measure an individual's health status.

A number of empirical studies were reviewed. Some of the more important findings are the following: (1) The income elasticity with respect to medical care expenditures is less than one but the income elasticity with respect to dental care expenditures is greater than one; (2) the demand for health services is quite inelastic with respect to price; (3) persons with health insurance have higher out-of-pocket expenditures on health care than persons without insurance; and (4) the demand for health insurance is more elastic with respect to price than the demand for medical care services.

Notes

1. Richard H. Leftwich, *The Price System and Resource Allocation* (New York: Holt, Rinehart and Winston, 1960), p. 27.

2. Leftwich, *The Price System*, p. 28.

3. Alfred Marshall, *Principles of Economics*, (8th Ed.) (London, England: Macmillan and Co., Ltd., 1920), Bk. III, Chapter 10.

4. Engel curves are named after Ernst Engel, a German pioneer of the last half of the nineteenth century in the field of budget studies. See George J. Stigler, "The Early History of Empirical Studies of Consumer Behavior," *The Journal of Political Economy*, Vol. 62, April 1954, pp. 98-100.

5. Howard R. Bowen and James R. Jeffers, *The Economics of Health Services* (New York: General Learning Press, 1971), p. 8.

6. Irving Leveson, "The Demand for Neighborhood Medical Care," *Inquiry*, Vol. 7, No. 4, December 1970, p. 22.

7. Bowen and Jeffers, *The Economics of Health Services*, p. 8.

8. Commission on the Cost of Medical Care, *General Report*, Vol. I (Chicago, Illinois: American Medical Association, 1964), p. 59.

9. Grover C. Wirick, "A Multiple Equation Model of Demand for Health Care," *Health Services Research*, Winter, 1966, Vol. I, No. 3, p. 304.

10. Ibid.

11. Wirick, "A Multiple Equation Model of Demand," p. 305.

12. Hyman Joseph, "Empirical Research on the Demand for Health Care," *Inquiry*, Vol. 8, No. 1, March 1971, p. 62.

13. Milton Friedman and Simon Kuznets, *Income from Independent Professional Practice* (New York: National Bureau of Economic Research, 1945), pp. 157-58.

14. Joseph, "Empirical Research," p. 62.

15. Milton Friedman, *A Theory of the Consumption Function* (Princeton, New Jersey: Princeton University Press, 1967).

16. Feldstein and Carr obtained an elasticity estimate for total medical expenditures, including insurance, in 1950 of 0.5 for measured income and 1.0 for permanent income. See Paul Feldstein and John Carr, "The Effect of Income on Medical Care Spending," *Proceedings of the Social Statistics Section of the American Statistical Association*, Vol. 7, 1964, pp. 95, 100 and 101.

17. See Victor R. Fuchs, "Some Economic Aspects of Mortality in the United States," unpublished manuscript, National Bureau of Economics Research, July

1965; and Richard Auster, Irving Leveson, and Deborah Sarachek, "The Production of Health: An Exploratory Study," *Journal of Human Resources*, Vol. 4, Fall, 1969, pp. 411-36.

18. Irving Leveson, "The Demand for Neighborhood Medical Care," p. 21.

19. Grover C. Wirick and Robin Barlow, "The Economic and Social Determinants of the Demand for Health Services," in *The Economics of Health and Medical Care* (Ann Arbor, Michigan: The University of Michigan, 1964), pp. 95-125.

20. Wirick and Barlow, "Economic and Social Determinants," p. 123.

21. George J. Stigler, *The Theory of Price* (New York: Macmillan, 1952), p. 75.

22. U.S. Department of Health, Education and Welfare, Public Health Service, Health Resources Administration, *Expenditures for Personal Health Services: National Trends and Variations, 1953-1970* (Washington, D.C.: U.S. Government Printing Office, 1973), p. 6.

23. Herbert E. Klarman, *The Economics of Health* (New York: Columbia University Press, 1965), p. 35.

24. Joseph, "Empirical Research," p. 65.

25. Victor Fuchs and Marcia Kramer, *Determinants of Expenditures for Physicians' Services in the United States, 1948-1968* (New York: National Bureau of Economic Research, Occasional Paper 117, 1974), p. 34.

26. Michael Grossman, *The Demand for Health: A Theoretical and Empirical Investigation* (New York: National Bureau of Economic Research, Occasional Paper 119, 1972), p. XVI.

27. Ronald Anderson and Lee Benham, "Family Income and Medical Care Consumption," in Herbert E. Klarman (Ed.), *Empirical Studies in Health Economics* (Baltimore, Maryland: The Johns Hopkins Press, 1970), p. 92.

28. Gerald Rosenthal, "Price Elasticity of Demand for Short-Term General Hospital Services," in Herbert E. Klarman (Ed.), *Empirical Studies in Health Economics* (Baltimore, Maryland: The Johns Hopkins Press, 1970), p. 104.

29. Rosenthal, "Price Elasticity of Demand," p. 114.

30. Victor Fuchs, "Comment" (Rosenthal's paper) in Herbert E. Klarman (Ed.), *Empirical Studies in Health Economics* (Baltimore, Maryland: The Johns Hopkins Press, 1970), p. 119.

31. Ibid.

32. Hyman Joseph, "Hospital Insurance and Moral Hazard," *Journal of Human Resources*, Vol. 7, No. 2, Spring, 1972, p. 156.

33. Joseph, "Empirical Research," p. 159.

34. Cited in Charles E. Phelps, "The Demand for Reimbursement Insurance," paper presented at the National Bureau of Economic Research Conference on Health Insurance and Medical Care, May 30-June 1, 1974, p. 36.

35. Phelps, "The Demand for Reimbursement Insurance," p. 34.

36. Paul J. Feldstein, *Financing Dental Care: An Economic Analysis* (Cambridge, Massachusetts: Heath Lexington, 1973), p. 37.

37. Charles Upton and William Silverman, "The Demand for Dental Services," *Journal of Human Resources*, Vol. 7, No. 2, Spring, 1972, pp. 250-61.

38. Leveson, "The Demand for Neighborhood Medical Care," p. 19.

39. Jan Paul Acton, *Demand for Health Care When Time Prices Vary More Than Money Prices*, R-1189-OEOINYC (Santa Monica, California: The Rand Corporation, May 1973), p. 17.

3 Health Manpower

This chapter focuses on a variety of dimensions of the health manpower problem. Consideration is given to techniques of manpower projection, the use of medical auxiliaries in rich and poor nations, the severity of the doctor shortage (as well as other health personnel) in the United States, the maldistribution of physicians, and the problems associated with the emigration of health professionals to the United States.

Health Manpower Projections

The aim of manpower projections is to provide a quantitative assessment of the balance between future manpower requirements and supplies. This involves the preparation of separate projections of requirements and supplies so that the disparity, if any, between them can be determined.

The first step in supply analysis is to decide whom to include. Doctors, nurses, dentists, technicians, and pharmacists should be counted. Midwives, herbalists, and similar categories should be included where they are numerically important. It is not generally necessary to count untrained persons who are employed by medical institutions. Most ambulance drivers, hospital maids, and hospital clerks should not be included as they are a part of larger general manpower pools.[1]

Supply is partly determined by the number of training institutions that provide new entrants into the occupation as well as by the total number of new applicants. If training facilities are limited, entry into the field may be restricted. Licensure, another supply component, effectively controls entry into the medical profession. While in some cases it protects the consumer from incompetent health personnel, it has frequently acted as an important barrier to entry especially in the nursing and dental fields.[2]

There are several factors that reduce the supply of health personnel. The first is losses due to death. However, retirement is usually the greatest source of reduction in the number of health workers. In some countries losses caused by change of occupation are very significant. For example, in most of Latin America, where the medical degree is often the mark of the educated person, many physicians do not practice medicine.[3] In the United States it is estimated that almost 500,000 registered nurses and licensed practical nurses are currently inactive.[4] Finally, the last major source of losses (gains) to the medical

41

profession is through migration. Moreover, if a professional from a developing country undertakes a 10 year course of study in a highly specialized field of medicine that is irrelevant to the health problems of his own nation, he is essentially as much of a "loss" to his profession as the individual who migrates.

A number of methods are utilized to project requirements for health manpower. One of the more traditional approaches is the physician population ratio. This approach assumes that the present ratio of doctors (or nurses or x-ray technicians) to the population is the adequate requirement. Future requirements for doctors are simply the expected future population times the present doctor/population ratio. A number of criticisms have been made of this approach. First, it ignores changes in population composition, thereby disregarding each population subgroup's differing medical demands. Moreover, this method does not consider possible changes in the productivity of health personnel as well as the possibility of substituting one type of medical personnel for another.[5]

Another approach is through projecting current physician utilization rates into the future, keeping them constant for each socioeconomic-demographic population group. The entire change in utilization is thus attributed to changes in the number and composition of the population.

However, patterns of per capita use may change over time. If data are available for more than a single period, past trends can be projected into the future. Above all, it is desirable to obtain patterns of utilization for the population classified according to as many different characteristics as possible.

A third method is to project expenditures for a particular type of service, such as physicians' visits or dental care. This is usually done by means of regression analysis.

Manpower requirements are then derived by (a) projecting annual expenditures per provider of services, or by (b) examining the effect on prices and providers' income of the calculated gap between projected supply and projected demand. In either case it is necessary to deal explicitly with the providers' earnings. The second method also involves consideration of the price elasticity of demand.[6]

How accurate are physician manpower projections? Table 3-1 summarizes the results of a number of studies that developed physician projections for 1975 based on a number of approaches.

Although the magnitudes of the deficits differ a great deal, it is clear that most of the projections forecast a deficit of physicians in 1975. However, it should be noted that these projections imply a shortage of health manpower that may be overstated. This is because they do not consider the potential flexibility in the production of health services. For example, physicians may make increasing use of nurses and assistants. Similarly, drugs and other new treatments can be substituted for more traditional treatment regimens that require far more physician time. Given these substitution possibilities and the failure to incorporate them into projections, it is little wonder that such exercises have been generally viewed with scepticism.

Table 3-1
Summary of Physician Projections for 1975

Projection study	Requirements	Supplies	Surplus or Deficit
Perrott-Pennell (1958)	301,370[a]	290,409	−10,961
	325,139[b]	293,382	−31,757
Bane Report (1959)	330,000	312,800[c]	−17,200
		318,400[d]	−11,600
Bureau of Labor Statistics (1967)	360,000	390,000	+30,000
Public Health Service (1967)	400,000[e]	360,000	−40,000
	425,000[f]		−65,000
Fein (1967)	372,000-385,000	361,700	−10,300 to −23,300
National Advisory Commission on Health Manpower (1967)	346,000	360,000	+14,000

[a]Maintain 1955 physician population ratio.

[b]Increase graduates sufficiently to maintain 1955 ratio of graduates to population 20-24 years of age.

[c]Increase graduates to maintain 1957 physician population ratio.

[d]Raise those states below average to 1957 population ratio.

[e]Based on application of professional standards.

[f]Applies the highest physician utilization rate among the four major regions of the United States to the entire 1975 population.

Source: W. Lee Hansen, "An Appraisal of Physician Manpower Projections," *Inquiry* Vol. VII, No. 1, March 1970, p. 107; Irene Butter, "Health Manpower Research—A Survey," *Inquiry*, Vol. 4, No. 4, December 1967, p. 16; David Bergwall, Philip N. Reeves, and Nina B. Woodside, *Introduction to Health Planning* (Washington, D.C.: Information Resources Press, 1974), p. 147.

Moreover, recent statistics indicate that the majority of the supply projections presented in Table 3-1 were too low. The 1973 American Medical Association (AMA) census of physicians indicates that there were 366,000 physicians practicing in the United States during that year, an increase of 10,000 over 1972.[7] Thus, by 1975 (the end of the year projection) there will be nearly 390,000 physicians in the United States.

Is There a Physician Shortage?

A shortage of medical care services can arise if, at current medical care prices and at current incomes, individuals demand medical care but find that the desired services cannot be obtained. This situation involves a "shortage" based on an economic rather than a medical need criterion. Such a shortage can occur if prices are inflexible, that is, not affected by changes in supply or demand. Moreover, if prices rise too slowly to clear the market, a shortage may occur. In addition, various parts of the medical care field are characterized by restrictions on entry. Thus, the supply of services is less than potential providers could make available. Prices therefore can be maintained above competitive levels. In a sense, this is also a shortage. While not visible, it nonetheless exists.[8]

There are a variety of methods that have been used to determine the magnitude of the physician shortage. In the classic 1933 monograph by Roger I. Lee and Lewis W. Jones, the estimate of *need* was based on a consensus of expert opinion regarding the amount of care, that is, the number of physician hours required to prevent, diagnose, and treat specific diseases and health conditions. The study translated the number of hours needed into a physician requirement: 134.7 physicians per 100,000 population (about 165,000 physicians for the nation).[9] The 1930 census listed 154,000 active physicians. Not all of these physicians, however, were available for full-time patient care. Thus, using the criteria developed by Lee and Jones, there was a shortage of physicians.

The relating of morbidity to hours of treatment was a major step forward as compared to the more usual process of relating numbers of physicians to population. Morbidity rates change, however, as do the number of hours needed to treat a particular condition.[10]

This approach has recently been replicated in a study by Hyman K. Schonfeld, Jean F. Heston and Isidore S. Falk, which estimated the number of physicians (pediatricians and internists) required for primary medical care. They found that primary medical care of good quality requires the services of about 133 physicians per 100,000 persons of all ages in the population. For a current total population of about 200 million, this means about 266,000 physicians are needed for primary medical care. According to the authors there were only 59 primary care physicians per 100,000 in 1970, indicating a severe shortage of primary care medical practitioners.[11]

Rashi Fein has clearly stated the problems with this approach. First it assumes that people are able to pay for the medically desirable quantity of physicians' services.

Thus, even where there are a sufficient number of services or physicians available, many persons would still be deterred by a shortage of money from utilization of medical services. . . . Secondly, in establishing the "required" number of physicians—with requirements based on "optima" rather than averages—it should be recognized that some individuals will use services less frequently than others. Again, the fact that physicians are available does not mean that they will be utilized to advantage by various parts of the population. . . . Finally, there is the question of the priority to be accorded health care given the fact that there are scarce resources. While professional standards are valuable as guidelines they cannot serve as absolutes. They do not replace the need for allocation decisions by those who must view the competing demands of the various sectors: health education, pollution control, housing, etc. These decisions will always be required.[12]

The Relative Income Method

This approach, first utilized by David S. Blank and George J. Stigler, indicates that in an economy with a free labor market there is evidence of a shortage when the salaries in the occupation under consideration increase more rapidly than in comparable occupations.[13] For example, from 1959-69 the median earnings of physicians increased from $22,100 to $40,550, an increase of 87 percent.[14] In contrast the median earnings of all male professional and technical workers increased from $6,622 to $10,617, an increase of 61 percent.[15] Moreover, the rate of increase in physicians' incomes was considerably greater than that of earnings of workers in service or manufacturing industries. This implies according to the Blank and Stigler criteria that the shortage of physicians worsened during the 1960s.

Two objections to this approach are that the lag in adjustment to dynamic changes in demand is not considered and that neither the beginning nor direction of the shortage is directly ascertainable.

Another weakness with the above method is that it does not consider the cost of training. An investment concept known as the internal rate of return considers both the costs of training and the economic returns that accrue to individuals who have obtained training. This figure can be found by calculating the rate of discount that equates the present value of the expected earnings stream to the present value of the expected outlay or cost stream. This amounts to viewing training as an investment in human capital that yields a continuing flow of money returns.

According to W. Lee Hansen's calculations, the internal rate of return for medical education fell from 13.4 percent in 1949 to 12.8 percent in 1956[16]—this compared with a return of 11.5 percent and 11.6 percent for male college graduates for the same years. Thus, Hansen concluded that the degree of shortage of physicians had been declining, or, in other words, that the magnitude of underinvestment in training for the medical profession had diminished. However, more recent studies imply a sharp increase in the rate of return to medical education. Frank A. Sloan found that the rate of return increased from 14.7 percent in 1959 to 18.2 percent in 1966.[17] Fein and Gerald I. Weber calculated a return of from 15 to 18 percent.[18] This is considerably higher than the unadjusted return to schooling for male college graduates, which falls between 10 and 12 percent. This implies that the shortage of physicians worsened during the 1960s.

Another method of determining shortages is to survey institutions that employ health manpower and for each of a variety of occupations determine the number of current vacancies as well as the number of additional workers needed because of personnel turnover and organizational expansion. For example, one widely quoted estimate indicated a shortage of 50,000 physicians in the United

States. How was this figure derived? Those who made the estimate observed that group practice physicians could provide comprehensive care at the rate of 100 physicians per 100,000 population. Using this ratio they determined that 27 states had fewer than 100 physicians per 100,000 population. When one applied this ratio nationally, the inference was a need for 12,000 additional physicians.[19]

A federal agency, the Office of Economic Opportunity, was asked what its requirements were for staffing 800 community health centers, each of which would serve 10,000 people. The estimate was that 10 physicians would be required for each center. This implied a need for 8,000 physicians to provide care in urban ghettos and other areas. Psychiatric services are also felt to be in short supply and the National Institute of Mental Health determined that at least 15,000 additional psychiatrists are needed. Data published by the American Medical Association implied that 10,000 additional physicians are needed to fill internships and residencies in approved programs. Finally, there was an expressed need for 5,000 additional physicians in teaching, research, and administration, including 1,700 medical school faculty positions that were budgeted but not filled.[20]

While this approach may be useful, one should not expect good results unless the demand for and supply of medical personnel are fairly stable. The demand for auxiliary personnel in physicians' offices, for example, will not be measured accurately by asking physicians about manpower needs if there is a large rate of increase in doctors.[21] Moreover, the local dentist's projected hiring of another dental hygienist two years from now assumes that dental hygienists' wages will not rise too much in the intervening period; but if all dentists expect to hire a hygienist, wages will rise substantially and expected hirings will not occur.

Fein used the "constant utilization rates for a changed population" approach discussed earlier. He did not attempt to estimate the magnitude of the physician shortage but instead tried to determine whether or not it would become worse. Recognizing that different race, age, sex, education, income, and regional groups exhibit different needs or utilize doctors' services differently, he estimated physician requirements for each group separately, then added up separate demands to get an overall figure.

Fein's results indicated that physician visits will increase by between 22 and 26 percent between 1965 and 1975.[22] Of this, 12 to 15 percent (about 4/7 of this projected increase in demand) is accounted for by growth of the total population. Thus, about 3/7 of the growth in demand is due to other quantifiable factors that would have been ignored in the more traditional aggregated simple population-ratio requirement projections. Fein expected that the supply of physicians would increase by 19 percent or about 3 to 7 percent less than the demand for physicians' services. Thus, in the absence of productivity and organizational change within the health care system, he expected the shortage of physicians to grow worse from 1965 to 1975.

Physician Productivity

Most observers are agreed that in the past there have been significant increases in the productivity of physicians as measured by the number of visits of constant quality per physician. Herbert E. Klarman summarizes the findings: Frank Dickenson's estimates for the 1940-50 decade range between 33 and 50 percent. Joseph Garbarino estimates a gain of 10 percent in the 1949-54 period. Richard Bailey estimates a 3.3 percent a year gain between 1949 and 1959, and Norman Jones estimates an increase of from 3.5 to 4.2 percent per year from 1960 to 1965.[23] The magnitude of future productivity gains is unpredictable. Productivity increases would permit the same services to be offered with fewer physicians or permit the same number of physicians to offer more services. This is of major importance since a 4 percent increase in the productivity of physicians would contribute more to augmenting the supply of health services than the annual number of medical school graduates from United States medical schools.

It has been suggested that improvements in the productivity of physicians may be more difficult to achieve in the future than it was in the past. Reduction in travel by physicians on home calls and in time per patient visit may have gone as far as possible without realizing adverse effects. In the future, gains in productivity may be expected from changes in the form of medical care organization, more institutional care, more automation and greater use of auxiliary health personnel.[24]

One of the means by which productivity of physicians may be increased is through group practice. Milton Roemer defines *group practice* as "three or more physicians of different specialties working together at one location and sharing income according to some prearranged plan."[25] There are several reasons why group practice can result in higher physician productivity. First, it is often found that larger organizational units are able to achieve economies that do not occur in those of smaller size. These economies of scale result from the fact that certain divisions of labor and specialization are made possible and justified when the number of units produced—or services rendered—is sufficiently large. Furthermore, various types of equipment and personnel are often available in "lumpy" units—one cannot buy half a machine or readily hire half a person. Thus, such equipment and personnel are used more efficiently in larger size production units. Since medical care involves the physician as well as other personnel and capital equipment, it is unlikely that the *optimal* combination of factors is likely to be found in the solo practitioner's office. These factors— physician, nurse, equipment, etc.—could only be utilized efficiently in whole unit relationships to each other, for example, one physician per one (or two or three, but not three-quarters or 1.2) x-ray machine.[26]

The inflexibility that exists in solo practice may have various consequences. Physicians may do without some equipment or personnel that would be useful. Thus, the physician would be operating below his potential level of efficiency.

Alternatively, physicians may purchase more equipment or employ more personnel than is needed. This is likely to result in higher cost of medical care since all patients will share in paying for the inefficiency.

The more effective use of personnel would permit a savings of physician's time and allow him to concentrate on those tasks for which he is uniquely qualified. If physicians are providing services that do not require the special skills of a physician, group practice can provide an organizational framework that makes it easier for other personnel to offer those services. Moreover, the training of such personnel is more readily achieved in the context of larger organizational structures.

However, recent empirical studies do not support the claim that group practice increases physician productivity. Richard Bailey found no difference in the productivity of physicians (as measured by office visits) between solo practitioners and group practices of varying sizes.[27] Moreover, he finds that the addition of paramedical personnel does not directly affect physician productivity but may result in the substitution of paramedical time for physician time spent on certain tasks that are extraneous to patient visits.[28] There may be several explanations for his finding of constant returns to scale. The one Bailey finds most satisfactory relates to medical training itself. "Group as well as nongroup physicians receive the same type of training in which the concept of following accepted patterns of health care is instilled in them. Group practice apparently does little to change these concepts."[29]

Joseph Newhouse argues that there are disincentives to work in many group practices that should be expected to reduce efficiency. Cost and revenue sharing schemes are more prevalent as group size increases; therefore, any individual physician is less likely to have to bear the financial consequences of his decision. Moreover, the financial reward he obtains from additional work effort falls. One would also expect that hours worked would fall as the physician's share of marginal revenue falls. Both Bailey and Newhouse find this prediction to be confirmed. Group practice reduces hours of work and thus in effect diminishes the supply of physician services.[30] Newhouse indicates that whatever economies of scale exist for group practice are exhausted so quickly (three or four physicians), that little emphasis should be placed upon them.[31]

A group practice that provides peer review may improve the quality of physician services and thus indirectly increase productivity. Eliot Friedson and Buford Rhea have reported that 33 percent of the physicians in 243 large group practices surveyed reported at least daily consultations with other physicians concerning patient treatment, while 27 percent reported such consultations only once or twice a week.[32] Peterson compared solo practitioners in North Carolina to physicians practicing in arrangements of two or more physicians. The physicians in partnership or group practice ranked higher in terms of qualitative criteria employed.[33] However, whether this was due to the pressure of peer review or the selection procedures used in forming the groups is impossible to determine.

Maldistribution of Health Manpower

Although the magnitude and severity of the physician shortage is controversial there is general agreement that health manpower is distributed very unevenly throughout the population. On a national basis there is one physician for 750 people. However, there are enormous variations in the ratio of health manpower to population by geographic areas. For example, in parts of Appalachia there is one physician for 5,000 to 10,000 persons. Massachusetts has a ratio of 18 doctors per 10,000 people compared with 7 per 10,000 in Mississippi. The District of Columbia has 32 physicians per 10,000 people but in Anacostia, a black community in northeast Washington, the ratio is 3 physicians per 10,000 residents.[34] In 1968 dentist to population ratios ranged from one dentist for every 3,726 persons in South Carolina to 1 for every 1,230 persons in New York State. The national average was 1 to 1,824.[35]

More physicians are tending toward a hospital-based practice as compared with an office-based practice. The hospital-based physician is most likely a specialist living in a metropolitan area where the large hospitals are located. The distribution of health manpower is related to the racial and socioeconomic changes in metropolitan areas. Shortages are particularly acute in rural areas and in poor urban communities. Manpower legislation has attempted to correct the problem by using incentives to encourage physicians to practice in these areas. The federal government will assume as much as 85 percent of the medical educational loans of physicians who elect to practice in either area. In order for these physicians to keep up with new trends in medical education, the legislation also provides for postgraduate centers for continuing study. In an investigation of 11 relatively limited state programs to encourage the movement of manpower to shortage areas, an average of 60 percent of the physicians "paid back" their loans by rural practice. However, in only one state, Kentucky, where 98 percent paid back their loans this way, did the number exceed two-thirds. Moreover, of five states with programs no longer in existence, only in Mississippi did a majority of physicians settle in rural areas.[36]

Gaston V. Rimlinger and Henry B. Steele found that high-income areas have substantially larger numbers of physicians in relation to population than low-income areas. This was because in high-income areas persons tend to visit physicians more often and have more expensive visits; furthermore, physicians were able to charge higher fees to higher income clients.[37]

As pointed out by Fein and Weber there is a chronic tendency for many states to underinvest in medical education because the states that export physicians are reluctant to expand facilities if a majority of their students will practice elsewhere. Moreover, states such as California and Florida, which receive a large number of physicians trained elsewhere, have very little incentive to expand medical school enrollment.

The primary factor affecting the location of new physicians is population change. Rapidly expanding states attract new physicians whether or not they are training them. States that have many graduates relative to their population find that a large proportion of their graduates migrate to other states.[38] The number of graduates from medical schools in a state does effect the number of physicians practicing in that state, but only 43 percent of the physicians in 1967 in each state received their medical school education in the state in which they were practicing. There is a very close relationship between the number of physicians per capita and the number of interns and residents per capita.[39] This suggests that if a state or particular area wishes to improve its per capita share of physicians it should make efforts to provide more internship and residency programs.

Allied Health Manpower

The health care industry in 1960 was recognized as the third largest in the United States, employing 4 percent of the civilian labor force (2.6 million). By 1970 the industry had increased employment to about 4 million up 56 percent (or 1.4 million) from the level 10 years earlier.[40] Since the beginning of the century the supply of health manpower has increased tenfold.[41] Slightly more than three-fourths of the growth during the 1960s was concentrated among allied health personnel reflecting the rapid increase in medical technology and the concomitant development of many new health care occupations to assist and extend the services rendered by the physician. Moreover, these workers are meeting with increased acceptance by the established health professions as well as greatly increased employment opportunities resulting from the sharp increase in the demand for health care. Between 1960 and 1970 the allied work force rose from 1.5 to 2.6 million (an increase of 75 percent), compared with a gain among health professionals of about 30 percent (from 1.0 to 1.3 million).

What is *allied health manpower*? The federal government considers this term to cover all health occupations below the doctoral level. "Allied health manpower, when used broadly, covers all those professional, technical, and supportive workers in the fields of patient care, community health, public health, environmental health, and health related research who engage in activity that supports, complements, or supplements the professional function of administrators, physicians and dentists."[42]

The terms used to describe the various allied health occupations and allied health personnel present several difficulties. For some fields the word "technologists" is used to mean a person with baccalaureate level preparation and the term "technician" refers to an individual with one or two years preparation. There are exceptions to this usage, and at the present time, there is lack of general agreement as to the educational qualifications that differentiate between technologists and technicians. In similar fashion the word "therapist" may denote a wide range of educational levels. A physical therapist has a baccalaure-

ate degree; an inhalation therapist often receives one year of technical preparation. An "assistant" is another word that in some fields means one or two years
of posthigh school preparation, in others a baccalaureate degree.[43]

At the present time there are approximately 300,000 allied health professionals (these are workers who have earned a minimum of a baccalaureate
degree). However, more attention should perhaps be given to the 1.7 million
nonprofessional allied health personnel. These workers appear to have several
common features. None has completed a four-year college education, which
places them in either the health technician or health assistant position. While
some of these individuals have received college training or an associate arts
degree, the majority are high school graduates who have received some type of
on-the-job training or training in a vocational school.

The health industry has some manpower characteristics that are very different
from other industries. For example, 70 percent of health workers are women
(and in the hospital setting, the ratio is three to one). Moreover, 40 percent of all
women workers in the health field are under the age of 35 years. This means that
many will leave the work force for varying periods in order to marry and raise a
family. This in part accounts for the high turnover rate among health workers. In
the technician and assistant category, four out of every five workers are women.

For health professionals, the overall supply of active workers is projected to
increase from 1.3 million in 1970 to 1.8 million in 1980, and to 2.2 million in
1990. (See Table 3-2.) This represents a gain of 66 percent over the 20 year
period, or an average annual rate of growth compounded of 2.6 percent—about
the same as that registered between 1960 and 1970. The gain in the first 10
years (1970-80) is expected to be somewhat faster than in the second 10 years
(1980-90), for health professionals as a group as well as for individual fields. The
fastest rate of growth is for registered nurses with the slowest growth occurring
among pharmacists.

Additional projections have been developed for a number of allied health
occupations. (See Table 3-3.)

According to the Department of Health, Education and Welfare (HEW), the
supply of allied health workers will fall nearly 25 percent short of the 1,776,000
needed by 1980. It has also been estimated that by 1980 the demand for health
workers requiring less than a college degree will be 580,000. However, a supply
of only 475,000 workers is projected. Thus, better utilization of the current
supply or innovative new patterns of manpower utilization must be developed.[44]

Severe shortages will also likely occur in dentistry. It is estimated that by
1980 there will be a need for 250,000 dental hygienists, assistants, and
technicians, but only 180,000 are expected to be available. The increased
emphasis on environment and pollution will also create a scarcity of environmental health workers. It is expected that approximately 155,000 workers in the
environmental health field will be required by 1980, about 65,000 more than
the supply.[45]

Table 3-2
Projected Supply of All Active Health Professionals, Actual 1960 and 1970, and Projected 1975-90

Year	All Health Professionals	Physicians (M.D.'s and D.O.'s) Combined	Dentists	Registered Nurses	Optometrists	Pharmacists	Podiatrists	Veterinarians
				Number Active				
1960	1,029,620	251,900	90,120	527,000	16,100	117,800	7,000	19,700
1970	1,328,520	323,200	102,220	723,000	18,200	129,300	7,100	25,500
1980	1,765,970	424,200	126,170	993,000	20,900	149,400	8,100	35,200
1990	2,205,310	562,400	154,910	1,215,000	16,500	187,900	12,600	46,000
				Percent Distribution				
1960	100	24.5	8.8	51.2	1.6	11.4	0.7	1.9
1970	100	24.3	7.7	54.4	1.4	9.7	0.5	1.9
1980	100	24.1	7.2	56.5	1.2	8.5	0.5	2.0
1990	100	25.5	7.0	55.1	1.2	8.5	0.6	2.1

Source: Bureau of Health Manpower Education, *The Supply of Health Manpower, 1970 Profiles and Projections to 1990* (Washington, D.C.: U.S. Government Printing Office, 1972), p. 49.

Table 3-3
Allied Health Requirements and Supply, 1967, 1975, and 1980

		1967	1975	1980
Allied health—at least baccalaureate:				
medical allied manpower	Requirement	225,000	— — —	— — —
	Supply	175,000	270,000	320,000
	Deficit	50,000	— — —	— — —
Environmental health manpower	Requirement	105,000	135,000	155,000
	Supply	54,500	80,000	90,000
	Deficit	50,500	55,000	65,000
Allied health—less than baccalaureate:				
medical allied manpower	Requirement	336,500	— — —	— — —
	Supply	276,500	400,000	475,000
	Deficit	60,000	— — —	— — —
Dental allied manpower	Requirement	165,700	202,000	246,000
	Supply	137,000	139,000	151,000
	Deficit	28,700	63,000	95,000
Environmental health manpower	Requirement	20,000	35,000	50,000
	Supply	10,500	20,000	30,000
	Deficit	9,500	15,000	20,000

Source: U.S. Department of Health, Education, and Welfare, *Report to the President and to Congress*—The Allied Personnel Training Act of 1966 as Amended (Washington, D.C.: U.S. Government Printing Office, 1969), p. 35.

New and Changing Roles
in Health Manpower

The role of the traditional nurse is evolving into one of increased and more formalized responsibility for primary health care. These persons are trained to take histories, do physical examinations, make simple diagnoses, and treat a limited number of conditions.[46] Studies have shown that 50 to 75 percent of a pediatrician's routine work could be very effectively delegated to others. It is estimated that by 1975, 8,000 to 12,000 pediatric nurse practitioners could be employed, a ratio of one pediatric nurse practitioner to every two pediatricians in the United States.[47] Moreover, a recent study by Alfred Yankauer and associates indicated that many tasks presently performed by obstetricians and gynecologists could be delegated effectively to nurses and that these physicians were willing to delegate this work to others.[48] B.D. Duncan and associates reviewed the medical charts of 182 children who were first examined by a pediatric nurse and subsequently by a pediatrician.[49] The pediatrician diagnosed a total of 278 conditions of which 239 were in total agreement with the nurses' findings. Of the 39 differences in diagnosis, 37 were judged not significant D.W. Schiff and associates studied the productivity of pediatric nurses trained in a University of Colorado program. After one was hired, the private practice of two pediatricians who both previously had full case loads increased by 18 percent.[50]

During the next 5 to 10 years, short-term programs, particularly those that accept registered nurses, will be the only important source of paramedics. Furthermore, because nurse practice laws are rather vague about the functions of a registered nurse, licensure problems for the pediatric nurse practitioner will be minimal.[51]

In the United States the concept of physician's assistant originated with the Armed Forces Medical Services. It was demonstrated that in one or two years it is possible to train young men with limited formal educations to become skilled medical corpsmen to screen patients, administer care, perform technical procedures, do intravenous transfusions, and perform other task-oriented procedures. To offset the shortage of physicians this concept is being transferred to the civilian community through physician's assistant training programs.

In 1970 the AMA's Council on Health Manpower recommended to the Board of Trustees the following working definition of the term *physician's assistant.* "The physician's assistant is a skilled person qualified by academic and practical training to provide patient services under the supervision and direction of a licensed physician who is responsible for the performance of that assistant."[52]

At present, there is no agreement on the best type of structure, curriculum, or format for the physician's assistant training program. The best known are the University of Washington's MEDEX program, and the physician's assistant program at Duke University. The MEDEX program recruits former military medics to train as physician's assistants. The men receive three months of intensive classroom training that emphasizes the areas of medicine in which the medical corpsmen have had relatively little exposure such as pediatrics or geriatrics.[53] The student MEDEX is then assigned to a general practitioner who serves as a preceptor for one year. The intent is that rural and inner city physicians will then hire MEDEX students on completion of their apprenticeship. Unfortunately, there is no published study that indicates the effectiveness of MEDEX graduates in increasing physician productivity.

Another approach used in educating the physician's assistant is that developed by Duke University. The program consists of a 24 month curriculum, which is divided into a 9 month didactic section and a 15 month clinical section. The original concept of the Duke program was to train physician's assistants to aid the general practitioner in community practices. However, as the program has become more sophisticated, the need for physician's assistants in more specific areas has been recognized. Consequently, the curriculum has been expanded to include clinical training directed toward pediatrics and surgery. The program's requirements are that the applicant have a minimum of a high school diploma with at least two science courses, a minimum of three years experience in the health care field with one year dealing with patient care, and demonstrated academic ability.[54] A study cited by Judith R. Lave, et al., of a general practitioner who hired a physician's assistant trained at Duke indicated that before the assistant was hired, the physician treated an average of 219 patients per week and spent an average of 9.85 minutes with each patient. During the two months after he hired the assistant, the physician treated 214 patients per week and spent an average of 5.6 minutes per patient; the assistant spent 5.8 minutes per patient and saved the physician about 43 percent of his time. In the same number of patient contact hours per week (36), the physician could have treated 76 percent more patients. Because he did not his net income declined, but the amount of his leisure time increased.[55]

One evaluation of the utilization of physician's assistants indicated that they were accepted by private practitioners but that there was some hostility in a hospital setting. As long as a physician (or a group of physicians) accepted full responsibility for a physician's assistant, organizational problems were minimal. However, there was no full-time medical staff in the hospital to accept the responsibility, and much confusion resulted as to his authorized tasks and appropriate relations with other health workers. Thus, full-time staff supervision by a physician appears to be required to successfully integrate a physician's assistant into the hospital staff.[56]

Richard Zeckhauser and Michael Eliastam, developed a production function that they have used to estimate the potential contribution of physician's assistants to the delivery of care in an urban health center. When taking on his most productive assignments, it is found that a physician's assistant can replace half of a full-time physician.[57] In the physician's assistant programs at Duke University, the average annual salary in 1973 had risen to $13,500. This is in rough accord with what the production function would have suggested: roughly one-half of the net incomes of physicians working in similar delivery modes.[58]

Health Manpower Legislation

By the early 1960s the need of federal aid for health professions education had become acute. While previously enacted legislation had authorized institutional grants to schools of public health for training purposes, nowhere in the statutes were there provisions for direct federal support of medical education and health manpower development per se.

The passage of the Health Professions Education Assistance Act of 1963 marked a major step forward. This law provided funds for school construction and student loans. Thus, $175 million was authorized for matching grants for construction to be given to schools training individuals for health careers at the professional level. The act permitted the grants to cover up to two-thirds of the cost of construction or major expansion.[59]

The student loan program provided for 90 percent federal contributions. Students could obtain loans of up to $4,000 a year, repayable within 10 years, beginning three years after graduation, to allow for internship and residency training.

The Allied Health Personnel Training Act of 1966 was passed by Congress in order to provide federal stimulus for increasing the supply of health manpower. The act authorized four types of grants to training centers for allied health professions. These included (1) construction of teaching facilities; (2) traineeships for advanced training of allied health professions personnel; (3) development of training methods for new types of health personnel; and (4) improvement grants to upgrade the quality of allied health curriculum. In 1968 the eligibility provisions were broadened to authorize grants to public or nonprofit agencies, institutions, organizations, as well as training centers.

Several important additions and modifications to federal programs supporting manpower training were included in the Health Manpower Act of 1968. Important changes in the construction program were the provision for aid to multipurpose facilities, and for increased federal matching from 50 to 66 2/3 percent in cases where a medical or nursing school is experiencing financial difficulties because of heavy expenses for projects such as major revisions in curriculum, replacement of obsolete facilities, or moving to a new location. Moreover, greater federal support was extended to schools of nursing, pharmacy, and veterinary medicine.

The student loan program was expanded. The funds available were increased from $25 million to $35 million but a reduction was made in the grace period for repaying loans except for students receiving advanced professional training.[60]

Upon signing the Comprehensive Health Manpower Training Act of 1971 and its companion measure the Nurse Training Act, former President Nixon said the two laws "constitute the most comprehensive health manpower legislation in the nation's history."

The 1971 act made clear that the federal government's primary interest is the production of health manpower professionals, an emphasis on people rather than buildings.[61] Thus, the program emphasizes per capita grants to health training institutions giving them an incentive to expand enrollment. This capitation program has replaced facilities construction as the number one fund provider for institutions. Moreover, an expanded system of scholarships and loans should increase the number of medical students from low socioeconomic groups. The act specifically authorizes assistance for the training of physician's assistants and nurse practitioners who intend to practice in areas where manpower shortages are most severe.

Thus, the Bureau of Health Manpower Education supports 39 programs to train physician's assistants in 26 states and the District of Columbia, involving about 1,440 students; 24 special projects to prepare nurse practitioners, involving 1,350 students; and 7 projects involving about 1,450 students learning to work as "expanded function auxiliaries" in dental care.[62] The 1971 Health Manpower Act also has various provisions authorizing programs to increase family practice physician training. During 1972 the Bureau of Health Manpower Education awarded more than $25 million for family medicine activities. This figure omits capitation grants that many schools will use for family medicine training.

Although the Nixon administration indicated that expansion of health manpower is a high priority item, the reality of the situation is that funding for this purpose showed little change between 1972 and 1974. (See Table 3-4.)

Health Manpower Planning in Developing Countries

Because of the severe shortage of health manpower in developing countries—a shortage that will last for many years—it is imperative that these nations plan effectively for the effective utilization and training of health manpower resources.

With the belief that health manpower planning must be undertaken on a scientific basis, the Department of International Health at the Johns Hopkins University has completed large-scale health manpower studies in Peru, Taiwan, and Turkey. As Carl E. Taylor and his colleagues have noted, a health manpower hourglass characterizes the profile of health occupations in most developing

Table 3-4
Federally Aided Health Training and Education (in Millions)

| | Outlays | | |
Degree or Certificate Training	1972 Actual	1973 Estimate	1974 Estimate
Degree or certificate training	802	999	983
Research personnel	121	106	94
Physicians	272	333	407
Dentists	60	79	85
Nurses	108	175	112
Mental health professionals	31	29	27
Other health professionals	92	144	139
Paramedical personnel	118	132	119
All other training	308	380	311
Total	1,110	1,379	1,293

Source: U.S. Bureau of the Budget, *Special Analyses: Budget of the United States Government, 1974* (Washington, D.C.: U.S. Government Printing Office, 1974), p. 144.

countries.[63] Physicians and specialists are at the upper end of the hourglass; a limited number of nurses and technicians constitute a slender neck; and the large base consists of herbalists, sagliks, curanderos, and other indigenous health workers. Focusing in depth upon different aspects of health manpower, a census of physicians and nurses was taken in each country. As expected, difficulties were encountered in obtaining reliable information about the gross income and fee schedule of physicians and a listing of the actual numbers of patients whom they regularly treated. In the absence of a complete inventory of doctors and nurses, both the tabular and cohort methods were used to determine supply. Trends in recruitment and admission policies of health training institutions, the design of curricula, and faculty staffing patterns were described for each country. In each study, problems were encountered in locating and defining sharply the number of health workers in the various manpower categories.

Taiwan, Turkey, and Peru have health problems that are similar to those in most developing nations. Infant and child mortality rates are high, infectious diseases such as tuberculosis are prevalent, and the population is increasing rapidly. The supply of physicians is inadequate and poorly distributed and physician productivity is low partly because of a lack of auxiliaries. In Taiwan and Peru a disproportionate number of physicians are in military service, leaving the civilian population poorly served. In Turkey and Peru scarce resources of skilled manpower are dissipated by very low rates of utilization; many physicians see only a few patients each day.[64] Medical schools are often overcrowded because they pursue an open admissions policy, and the teaching staff cannot do an effective job because classes are so large. As a result, the dropout rate is high. A large percentage of physicians from these countries emigrate to the United States, making the domestic shortage even more acute.

Each study developed a different technique for estimating the future demand and supply of health workers:

Peru

Thomas L. Hall relied on two methods in estimating future health manpower requirements. The first method was based on the concept of *rationalized demand*. This means that the demand for health manpower was disaggregated into as many different components as possible, with projections being made for each of these components. Then the reaggregation of the separate demands was undertaken in order to obtain a consolidated projection.[65] The second estimating method used in the Peruvian study was a *straight-line projection* that was used to estimate the demand for salaried personnel in private medical institutions. The projection considered staff-bed ratios, hospital discharge rates, and population growth trends.

The concept of rationalized demand is similar to Frederick Harbisons' and

C.A. Myers' *target-setting approach* in which the goals for manpower are specified, comparisons for specific items are made, and the resultant estimates are converted into educational requirements.[66]

Turkey

The Turkish manpower study concentrated on *technically feasible demand* as well as demand based on economic factors. The former reflects the fact that what can be done in health care is often much less than what should be done. Often an important impediment to effective implementation of health programs is lack of technical knowledge as well as the lack of appropriate administrative machinery.[67] In the private sector, demand was based on per capita income and the physician-population ratio in various parts of the country.

The researchers relied on three straight-line projections of the supply of health manpower, which were (1) a supply-attrition model for physicians that considered the number of expected medical graduates as well as the number lost by death, inactivity, or emigration; (2) the supply and labor force participation rate of nurses; and (3) the current supply of midwives.

Taiwan

A model was developed to determine the relative contribution to the demand for health services of the following variables: population, income, age, education, morbidity, and sex. The major dependent variable was the number of full-time equivalent health personnel required to meet measured demand. Although this approach was used to estimate the future demand for physicians, straight-line projections based on population increase were the basis for estimating the demand for other types of health workers. This latter procedure is justified because "predictions based on the use of more time consuming methods would not have differed greatly in absolute numbers of health workers."[68]

Although the Taiwan study indicated that by 1983 the demand for physicians and dentists will exceed the supply by a considerable amount, there was expected to be a severe surplus of nurses. However, the authors asserted that there would still be a shortage of college graduate nurses due to the high dropout rate and small numbers trained.

All three health manpower studies made certain assumptions about the status quo. For example, it was assumed that no change would be made in the organization of health care or in the relative importance of several methods of financing, whether private practice, publicly supported or through voluntary insurance.

How might health manpower planning be further improved? One way might be to devise experimental methods to provide health services and evaluate these, rather than to conduct wide-ranging surveys of present conditions.[69] This approach could, for example, yield answers to basic questions about the population that could be served effectively by a multidisciplinary team of defined size. Computer simulation and systems analysis could assist in generalizing these findings.

Finally, while individual demand is primarily for curative services, a goal of higher social priority is to improve preventive services rather than to strengthen existing arrangements for curative medical care. To accomplish this goal investment in agriculture, road building and housing may be more effective than increasing the supply of health professionals.

Medical Auxiliaries in Developing Countries

There is a severe shortage of physicians throughout the world. There are approximately 1.5 million physicians to serve 3.5 billion persons, that is, one physician to every 2,500 people. However, 1.2 million of these physicians provide care to the 1 billion people in the developed world and only 300,000 physicians serve the 2.5 billion of the developing world. In developed countries each physician serves less than 1,000 people. In the developing world the ratio is one doctor for 8,000 persons.[70]

Moreover, within countries there is a severe maldistribution between urban and rural areas. In the developing nations where 70 to 95 percent of the population lives in rural areas, the maldistribution is as significant as the overall shortage. This is illustrated by Table 3-5, which shows for five countries the distribution of physicians between the capital city and the rest of the nation.

The purpose of the health auxiliary is to overcome shortages of personnel.

Table 3-5
Distribution of Physicians by Population

Country	Capital City		Rest of Country	
	% Physicians	% Population	% Physicians	% Population
Jamaica	70	26	30	74
Guatemala	82	15	18	85
Senegal	63	15	37	85
Thailand	60	8	40	92
Kenya	54	5	46	95

Source: N.R.E. Fendall, *Auxiliaries in Health Care: Programs in Developing Countries* (Baltimore, Maryland: Published by The Johns Hopkins Press for the Josiah Macy, Jr. Foundation, © 1972), p. 38.

The auxiliary is much nearer to the people he serves in thought, culture, and way of life than the physician. Because of this, he is more likely to be accepted by the local residents. Moreover, because of his limited education he is more content with a less sophisticated way of life and is more likely than a physician to remain in rural areas. He ameliorates both the shortage and maldistribution of health manpower and bridges the gap between the full-fledged health professional and those who are part of the traditional culture. Auxiliaries provide at a relatively low cost for a much more extensive outreach of services than would occur in their absence. They also prevent a waste of highly skilled professional talent being occupied on mundane and routine tasks, while seriously ill patients are neglected due to lack of time.[71]

The various categories of health auxiliaries are indicated in Table 3-6. Some of the common auxiliary categories are related to independent paramedicals and professionals by function and level of education. Nursing and maternal and child health auxiliaries are becoming more important because of the emphasis on family planning.[72] Let us focus on three of the most widely used types of health auxiliaries:

The Medical Assistant

The medical assistant must be capable of providing certain kinds of primary medical care. He must also be able to distinguish major and minor illnesses and refer the former to a physician. He has the additional function of being required to provide emergency medical care, and possibly to initiate antiepidemic measures.

The training of a medical assistant should be directly related to the common diseases that occur in the area. The treatment he provides should be based on effectiveness and should also consider safety and ease of administration. For example, the treatment of malaria can be limited to the dispensing of chloroquin, with instructions given to the medical assistant that if a case does not respond within 48 hours it must be referred to a physician.

Medical assistants make a major contribution to health manpower in Africa. (See Table 3-7.) Thus, in many of the above countries the number of medical assistants is greater than the number of physicians.

The Auxiliary Midwife Pediatrician

Maternal and child health services are far below the need for these services in the developing countries. Services are generally available for only 5 to 20 percent of the population. However, the pattern of services is similar to that in the developed countries. With a different approach more services could be made available to the rural population.

Table 3-6
Classification of Health Auxiliaries and Their Relation to Professionals

Function	Professional (Degree Course)	Level of Education	
		Middle Level (High School Plus Two or More Years Training)	Low Level (Elementary or Middle School With Up to One Year Training)
Medical care			
a. Independent responsibility for treatment	Physician	Feldsher (Russia) Licentiate (India & Pakistan) Behdar (Iran) Medical assistant (Pacific & Africa)	Dresser First aid men Medical corpsman (armed services)
b. Comprehensive care	Occasional physician	Health officer (Ethiopia)	Village health worker
c. Diagnostic and therapeutic specialties	Specialist	Technicians—laboratory, x-ray, physiotherapy, etc.	Technical assistants
Hospital nursing	Degree nurse	Diploma nurse Auxiliary nurse	Auxiliary nurse Ward helper
General public health	Public health physician Public health nurse	Health visitor Community nurse	Community nurse
MCH and obstetrics	Physician Midwife	Midwife Auxiliary nurse midwife	Auxiliary nurse midwife Village midwife (trained) Trained dai
Sanitation	Sanitary engineer	Sanitarian	Sanitary inspector
Specialized functions for mass diseases	Public health specialist	Malaria officers (upper echelon)	Malaria sprayers, etc. Vaccination Leprosy officers Sleeping sickness officer Tuberculosis health Visitors

Source: Carl E. Taylor, "Training Health Auxiliaries," paper presented to the East-West Center for Cultural and Technical Inter-Change Conference on Public Health Training and Education in Asian Countries, Honolulu, Hawaii, June 22, 1965.

Table 3-7
Medical Assistant and Physician Manpower, Selected African Countries, 1970

Country	Medical Assistants	Physicians
Botswana	54	41
Chad	56	59
Gambia	229	667
Ghana	96	19
Malawi	461	59
Mali	18	121
Rwanda	115	62
Southern Rhodesia	1,153	833
Sudan	631	985
Tanzania	745	598
Uganda	136	718
Zaire	368	1,065

Source: World Health Organization, *World Health Statistics Annual, 1970*, Vol. III, Health Personnel and Hospital Establishments (Geneva, Switzerland: World Health Organization, 1974), pp. 1-12.

The training of the auxiliary midwife would need to emphasize prenatal, postnatal, and child care to detect major abnormalities. Such cases could then be referred to professional and paramedical personnel. The auxiliary midwife could well be left to take care of the minor aspects of care and normal delivery. This is the case in Senegal where in 1962, of 550,183 outpatients under five years of age seen by physicians, only 12,322 were admitted to hospitals. An additional 463,352 were attended by auxiliaries on an outpatient basis.[73] Thus, in most cases diagnosis could easily be made by specially trained auxiliaries in an outpatient setting.

The Auxiliary Sanitarian

Many environmentally related diseases still persist in poor countries and contribute heavily to morbidity and mortality. Yet, environmental measures are not technically very difficult to introduce to the rural areas. These measures include the improvement of indigenous housing, the development of adequate waste disposal, accessible and clean water, food inspection, and garbage disposal. If funds are available, auxiliary sanitarians can provide most of these services.

Training of auxiliaries in some countries is usually undertaken in separate schools for each discipline. However, there is a movement towards the combining of training in one institute. The advantages of the comprehensive auxiliary training school are numerous. First, there are savings in capital and operating expenditures as well as utilization of instructors. Much of the content of the curricula is common to each training program such as general education, the biological sciences, nutrition, child care, and health education.

Auxiliary Training

Auxiliary training should be continuing and repetitive. Provisions for in-service training are particularly necessary and refresher courses are most important for those with a very limited amount of formal schooling.

The team concept of health center work is important in practice and therefore auxiliaries should be trained to work as a team. For example, a prototype approach developed at Gondar, Ethiopia, includes a team of three: a health officer, a middle-level doctor trained to emphasize preventive work; a community nurse; and a sanitarian. These personnel are trained together because they must work together.

The most important determinant of success in any auxiliary program is supervision. When auxiliaries are assigned to curative work, supervision by doctors is customary. However, preventive work is often not considered sufficiently important to merit the supervisor's attention. In the more isolated rural subcenters auxiliaries normally have both preventive and curative responsibilities and should be routinely visited at least once a week, with an established mechanism for patient referral in the intervals.

Secondly, auxiliaries should be full time and should receive an adequate salary. Money saved by paying minimal salaries and expecting the auxiliary to supplement income through private practice is poor economy. Effective supervision requires direct financial control. Salary control of auxiliaries is most important in public institutions, but even in private hospitals, auxiliaries are typically salaried.

Finally, a multiplicity of different types of auxiliaries interferes with efficiency. It is better to have a few categories of auxiliaries with their relative roles and relationships clearly defined and with minimal overlapping. The health services of some countries have employed many different kinds of auxiliaries, with new categories appearing before the training of competing groups is phased out. These changing patterns are unfair to the auxiliaries since consistent career development becomes impossible.[74]

The cost of training auxiliaries is far less than that for physicians and dentists. This is illustrated in Table 3-8, which indicates the training costs in Kenya during 1965 for a variety of health personnel.

As is evident above, extensive use of health auxiliaries permits considerable savings in training costs. Moreover, there is no world market for auxiliaries so that one does not have to consider the problem of international migration of paramedical manpower.

Table 3-8

Comparative Cost of Training Professional and Paramedical Health Personnel, Kenya, 1965

Category	Cost (U.S. $)
Physician	$22,000-$28,000
Nurse	$3,381
Sanitarian	2,946
Radiographer	1,576
Medical care auxiliary	2,890
Health or sanitary assistant	787
Nursing auxiliary	2,167
Laboratory auxiliary	4,007

Source: N.R.E. Fendall, *Auxiliaries in Health Care: Programs in Developing Countries* (Baltimore, Maryland: Published by The Johns Hopkins Press for the Josiah Macy, Jr. Foundation, © 1972), pp. 184-85.

Foreign Medical Graduates and the Brain Drain

One of every six physicians now practicing in the United States is a graduate of a medical school located outside the United States and Canada. If Canadian graduates are also included, the proportion of foreign medical graduates in the United States rises to almost one-fifth. Altogether there are more than 63,000 foreign trained physicians in the United States. (See Table 3-9.)

Table 3-9

Foreign Medical Graduates in the United States by Geographical Region of Graduation, 1970

Geographical Region	Foreign Medical Graduates	
	Number	Percent
Africa	1,126	1.8
Asia	21,002	33.1
Europe	24,756	39.1
North America (Canada)	6,174	9.7
Latin America	9,929	15.7
Oceania	404	0.6
Total	63,391	100.0

Source: Rosemary Stevens and Joan Vermeulen, *Foreign Trained Physicians and American Medicine*, Bureau of Health Manpower Education (Washington, D.C.: U.S. Government Printing Office, 1972), p. 104.

The number of foreign trained physicians in the United States has been increasing rapidly. Excluding Canadians, the number of foreign medical graduates in this country rose from 31,000 in 1963 to 57,000 in 1970—a net gain of 26,000 physicians in a seven-year period. (See Table 3-10.)

The contribution of foreign trained physicians to the United States has always been large. At least one American specialty, psychiatry, owes much of its development to those who immigrated before World War II. In terms of individual contributions to medical progress, foreign educated physicians are among the prominent teachers and researchers in most American universities.[75] By the 1960s, however, there was another stream of foreign medical graduates, brought in to staff hospitals rather than to engage in scientific research.

The influx of foreign trained physicians has occurred for a variety of reasons. First, as indicated previously, there is a shortage of physicians in this country. Given the present restrictions on admission to United States medical schools, the gap in physician supply can only be alleviated by permitting foreign medical graduates to practice in this country. Moreover, physicians' incomes in the United States are 10 to 20 times greater than in most developing countries. This provides a very strong incentive to emigrate to the United States. Finally, there are other factors that draw individual physicians to the United States, such as the chance to work with sophisticated equipment or the opportunity to practice in a major urban area.

Most foreign medical graduates begin working in this country as hospital employees. It is in the hospital that the shortage of physicians is most severe. At the end of 1970, 28,000 of the 63,000 physicians from foreign schools were working full time as interns, residents, or staff.[76] While constituting less than

Table 3-10
Physicians and Surgeons Admitted to the United States as Immigrants, 1901-71

Year	Number Admitted
1901-10	4,915
1911-20	3,905
1921-30	5,905
1931-40	5,644
1941-50	3,919*
1951-55	5,537
1956-60	8,516
1961-65	9,834
1966-71	20,676

*Does not include data for 1946-48.

Source: Computed from data contained in Rosemary Stevens and Joan Vermeulen, *Foreign Trained Physicians and American Medicine*, Bureau of Health Manpower Education (Washington, D.C.: U.S. Government Printing Office, 1972), p. 95.

one-fifth of all the physicians in this country, about one-third of all physicians in hospital-based practice are foreign medical graduates.

Applications to United States medical schools since World War II have consistently exceeded the number accepted by about two to one. In 1970-71, nearly 13,500 applicants were rejected from American medical schools. Paradoxically, a large number of these unsuccessful applicants have a much stronger premedical education than many of the foreign medical graduates who enter the United States as interns. Yet, at the internship level, there are presently two posts available for every American medical graduate. In short, there is an apparent bottleneck in undergraduate (M.D.) education.[77]

A major problem in the area of quality control of health care is the influx of foreign medical graduates who have not passed the examination given by the Educational Council for Foreign Medical Graduates (ECFMG) or who have passed the examination but have not obtained a permanent medical license. Many of these individuals are delivering patient care. Forty-three state medical licensure boards provide for the issuance of limited or temporary licenses than can be renewed indefinitely in some cases under a variety of regulations.[78]

Analysis of 1971 data compiled by the AMA indicates that of a total of 70,000 foreign medical graduates who had passed the ECFMG examination about 15 percent were not fully licensed nor in approved training programs. Nearly half of the latter (5,284 persons) reported their primary activity as direct patient care.[79] In addition, there are several thousand foreign medical graduates who are not even certified by the Educational Council for Foreign Medical Graduates, who constitute in effect, a medical underground.

In theory, one would expect that the influx of foreign trained physicians would alleviate to some extent the geographic maldistribution of physicians since they would be more likely to practice in areas where the shortage of physicians was most severe. Using data on doctor/population ratios, Irene Butter and Richard Schaffner have shown that, in fact, foreign medical graduates have *increased* the disparity in the availability of physicians' services among states and between urban and rural areas since they tend to settle in areas with at least an average relative number of United States trained doctors.[80] However, statistics also indicate that the interstate movement of foreign medical graduates shows a moderate trend toward relieving shortages.[81] Yet, this trend is not strong enough to counteract the geographic disparity that results from the initial location of foreign medical graduates entering the United States, and more important, the present geographic maldistribution of American doctors.

There is considerable variation in the emigration flows of physicians to the United States by country of last residence. James E. Jonish developed a log linear regression equation based on data from 48 countries.[82] The estimating equation and cross section results are indicated below:

$$\text{Ln } \overline{M} = \ln a + b_1 \ln \frac{S}{P} + b_2 \ln \frac{NG}{P} + b_3 \ln \frac{Y}{P} + b_4 \ln S$$

$$\text{Ln } \overline{M} = 0.727 + 0.52 \; 1n\frac{S*}{P} + 1.47 \; 1n\frac{NG}{P} - 0.474 \; 1n\frac{Y*}{P} + 0.4631 \; 1n \; S**$$

*Significant at 0.05 level.
**Significant at 0.01 level.

$\overline{M}$ = average annual physician immigration to the U.S., 1963-67

$\dfrac{S}{P}$ = 1965 physician-population ratio

$\dfrac{NG}{P}$ = 1960 new graduate physician-population ratio

$\dfrac{Y}{P}$ = 1965 income per capita in U.S. dollars

S = 1965 stock of physicians

The results indicate that the major determinant of physician emigration was the current stock of physicians in the country. The sign of the coefficient of income per capita suggests that migration to the United States will be greater the lower the per capita income is within the country of emigration. This is reasonable since income per capita may serve as a proxy for the effective demand for medical services. The variable, physicians per population unit, indicates that the greater the availability of physicians' services (supply), the greater is the flow to the United States.

On the basis of the cost of medical education in the United States, the direct educational resource savings obtained from the inflow of foreign medical graduates from 1956 to 1968 has been calculated to be $782 million.[83] This calculation is too low since it ignores the foregone earnings and the value of services that would have been obtained from increased numbers of individuals in American medical schools. Thus, the inflow of foreign physicians has afforded the United States a significant savings in current educational resources, and a considerable expansion of medical school facilities would be necessary to produce domestically the same output of physician manpower.[a]

The most fundamental reason for deterring emigration of medical personnel from developing countries is the severe shortage of physicians in these countries particularly in the rural areas. For example, some African countries have only one physician per 50,000 persons. As indicated above, most of the doctors are concentrated in the major urban centers leaving the rural areas virtually devoid

---

[a]If this calculation were made in terms of the costs incurred by the countries of origin in educating these physicians, the figure would be much lower. However, these latter costs would likely represent a larger fraction of the country's Gross National Product.

of physicians. Doctors would be more willing to accept positions in rural areas if they did not have the option of emigrating to a developed country. It seems absurd for the United States (as well as other developed countries) to be receiving such large scale "reverse foreign aid" because we are unwilling to train sufficient graduates of American medical schools.

There are two closely related suggestions that have been made to diminish the flow of foreign physicians to the United States. One is to indigenize foreign medical institutions. An essential part of this process would be to evolve local qualifications that were highly suitable to the medical needs of the local populace and relatively unacceptable to overseas employers. Thus, for instance, medical schools might graduate physicians who know a great deal about preventing the spread of tropical diseases and very little about curing the chronic diseases that are more common in the Northern hemisphere. Secondly, there is a close positive association between the rate of emigration to the United States from a particular country and the proportion of specialists trained in that nation.[84] These specialists tend to concentrate in urban areas of the developing countries where the effective demand for their services is low. Thus, because they are unable to earn a satisfactory income in their native land, they are likely to emigrate to developed countries. This pattern would perhaps be modified if medical schools concentrated on preparing their graduates for general practice.

Summary

A variety of methods including the "biologic demand" approach (Lee and Jones) and the "constant utilization rates for a changed population" approach (Fein) indicate that a doctor shortage exists in the United States. While productivity gains and the use of auxiliaries may narrow the gap between supply and demand for health services at constant prices, shortages of allied health manpower will limit the utilization of auxiliaries for the next 5 to 10 years. This implies that unless we increase medical school enrollments and economize on the use of available auxiliaries, this country faces a prolonged period of reliance on foreign medical graduates to meet a major part of our health needs.

There is a severe maldistribution of health manpower. A number of states as well as the federal government have passed laws designed to provide incentives for physicians to practice in areas of acute shortage. However, physicians tend to prefer practice in high income states with a rapidly expanding population.

Health manpower is in critically short supply in developing countries. Because of limited financial resources, health services can be extended to more individuals if a major effort is made to train health auxiliaries; especially medical assistants, auxiliary midwife pediatricians, and auxiliary sanitarians. In addition, greater efforts must be made in the area of manpower planning so that resources are allocated to the areas of greatest need. Finally, the emigration of health professionals should be discouraged, perhaps by indigenizing the medical school curriculum, or passing legislation in the developing countries designed to prevent or discourage the emigration of health professionals.

Notes

1. Timothy D. Baker, "Health Manpower Planning," in William A. Reinke (Ed.), *Health Planning: Qualitative Aspects and Quantitative Techniques* (Baltimore, Maryland: Waverly Press, 1972), pp. 180-81.

2. David F. Bergwall, Philip N. Reeves, and Nina B. Woodside, *Introduction to Health Planning* (Washington, D.C.: Information Resources Press, 1974), p. 139.

3. Baker, "Health Manpower Planning," p. 185.

4. U.S. Department of Labor, Manpower Administration, *Technology and Manpower in the Health Service Industry*, Manpower Research Bulletin, No. 14 (Washington, D.C.: U.S. Government Printing Office, 1967), p. 81.

5. Marsha Goldfarb, *A Critique of the Health Manpower Planning Literature*, Working Paper 73-2, Yale University School of Medicine, pp. 4-5.

6. Herbert E. Klarman, "Economic Aspects of Projecting Requirements for Health Manpower," *Journal of Human Resources*, Vol. 3, Summer, 1969, p. 365.

7. American Medical Association, *Research Notes*, Vol. 1, No. 1, August 1974, "AMA's Annual Study Describes Distribution of MD's in U.S.," p. 1.

8. Rashi Fein, *The Doctor Shortage: An Economic Diagnosis* (Washington, D.C.: The Brookings Institution, 1967), p. 16.

9. Roger I. Lee and Lewis W. Jones, *The Fundamentals of Good Medical Care* (Chicago, Illinois: University of Chicago Press, 1933), p. 115.

10. Fein, *The Doctor Shortage*, p. 7.

11. Hyman K. Schonfeld, Jean F. Heston, and Isidore S. Falk, "Number of Physicians Required for Primary Medical Care," *New England Journal of Medicine*, Vol. 286, No. 11, May 16, 1972, pp. 574-75.

12. Fein, *The Doctor Shortage*, pp. 7-8.

13. David S. Blank and George J. Stigler, *The Demand and Supply of Scientific Personnel* (New York: National Bureau of Economic Research, 1957), pp. 19-33.

14. U.S. Department of Health, Education and Welfare, *Medical Care Costs and Prices* (Washington, D.C.: U.S. Government Printing Office, 1972), p. 43.

15. U.S. Bureau of the Census, 1960 Census of Population, *Occupational Characteristics* (Washington, D.C.: U.S. Government Printing Office, 1973), Table 4, p. 145.

16. W. Lee Hansen, "Shortages and Investment in Health Manpower" in *The Economics of Health and Medical Care* (Ann Arbor, Michigan: University of Michigan School of Public Health, 1964), p. 86.

17. Frank A. Sloan, "Economic Models of Physician Supply," unpublished doctoral dissertation, Harvard University, 1968, p. 164.

18. Rashi Fein and Gerald I. Weber, *Financing Medical Education* (New York: McGraw Hill Book Co., 1971), p. 249.

19. E.A. Confrey, "The Logic of a Shortage of Health Manpower," *International Journal of Health Services*, Vol. 3, No. 2, 1973, p. 253.

20. Ibid.

21. Goldfarb, *A Critique*, p. 15.

22. Fein, *The Doctor Shortage*, p. 60.

23. Klarman, "Economic Aspects," p. 371.

24. Ibid., p. 370.

25. Milton I. Roemer, "Group Practice: A Medical Care Spectrum," *The Journal of Medical Education*, Vol. 40, No. 12, December, 1965, p. 1156.

26. Fein, *The Doctor Shortage*, pp. 97-98.

27. Richard Bailey, "Economics of Scale in Medical Practice," in Herbert E. Klarman (Ed.), *Empirical Studies in Health Economics* (Baltimore, Maryland: The Johns Hopkins Press, 1970), p. 268.

28. Bailey, "Economics of Scale," p. 270.

29. Ibid., p. 269.

30. Joseph Newhouse, "The Economics of Group Practice," Journal of Human Resources, Vol. 8, No. 1, Winter, 1973, p. 50. However, hours of work is a poor measure of productivity. Physicians' visits per hour or week is a better measure. Moreover, a productivity measure based on physician hours ignores the effects of ancillary personnel.

31. Newhouse, "The Economics of Group Practice," p. 45.

32. Eliot Friedson and Buford Rhea, "Physicians in Large Medical Groups: A Preliminary Report," *Journal of Chronic Diseases*, Vol. 17, September 1964, pp. 827-36.

33. Osler L. Peterson, Leon P. Andrews, Robert S. Spain, and Bernard G. Greenberg, "An Analytical Study of North Carolina Practice: 1953-1954," *Journal of Medical Education*, Vol. 31, No. 12, Part 2, December 1956, pp. 18-47.

34. James O. Hepner and Donna M. Hepner, *The Health Strategy Game: A Challenge for Reorganization and Management* (St. Louis, Missouri: The C.V. Mosby Co., 1973), p. 127.

35. American Dental Association, Bureau of Economic Research and Statistics, *Distribution of Dentists in the United States by State, Region, District and County*, 1969.

36. Henry R. Mason, "Effectiveness of Student Aid Programs Tied to a Service Commitment," *Journal of Medical Education*, Vol. 46, No. 7, July 1971, pp. 580-81.

37. Gaston V. Rimlinger and Henry B. Steele, "An Economic Interpretation of the Spatial Distribution of Physicians in the United States," *The Southern Economic Journal*, Vol. 30, No. 1, July 1963, pp. 1-12. A 1934 study by Leland

yielded similar conclusions. See R.G. Leland, *Distribution of Physicians in the United States*, Bureau of Medical Economics (Chicago, Illinois: American Medical Association, 1936).

38. Fein and Weber, *Financing Medical Education*, p. 178.

39. R.M. Scheffler, "The Relationship Between Medical Education and the Statewide Per Capita Distribution of Physicians," *Journal of Medical Education*, Vol. 46, No. 11, November 1971, p. 996.

40. Bureau of Health Manpower Education, *The Supply of Health Manpower, 1970 Profiles and Projections to 1990* (Washington, D.C.: U.S. Government Printing Office, 1972), p. 45.

41. Hepner and Hepner, *The Health Strategy Game*, p. 205.

42. "Personnel Training Act of 1966 as Amended," *Report to the President and Congress on the Allied Health Professions* (Washington, D.C.: U.S. Government Printing Office, 1969), p. 1.

43. *Report of the Allied Health Professions Education*, Subcommittee of the National Advisory Health Council to Education for the Allied Health Professions and Services (Washington, D.C.: U.S. Government Printing Office, 1970), p. 10.

44. Hepner and Hepner, *The Health Strategy Game*, p. 200.

45. Ibid.

46. Robert H. Drachman and Robert E. Cooke, "Physician Productivity and Medical Care," *The Journal of Pediatrics*, Vol. 77, No. 5, p. 757.

47. Hepner and Hepner, *The Health Strategy Game*, p. 221. However, it should be noted that a nurse and a pediatric nurse practitioner perform quite different tasks. In terms of training, one first becomes a nurse and after completing additional training is qualified for employment as a nurse practitioner.

48. Alfred Yankauer, Sally H. Jones, Jan Schneider, and Louis Hellman, "Performance and Delegation of Patient Services by Physicians in Obstetrics-Gynecology," *American Journal of Public Health*, August 1971, Vol. 61, No. 8, pp. 1545-1555.

49. B.D. Duncan, et al., "Comparison of the Physical Assessment of Children by Pediatric Nurse Practitioners and Pediatricians," (Colorado: University of Colorado, 1970), mimeographed.

50. D.W. Schiff, et al., "The Pediatric Nurse Practitioner in the Office of Pediatricians in Private Practice," *Pediatrics*, Vol. 44, July 1969, p. 62.

51. Judith R. Lave, Lester B. Lave, and Thomas E. Morton, "The Physicians' Assistant," *Hospitals*, Vol. 45, June 1, 1971, p. 44. The growth in the number of pediatric nurse practitioners will likely tend to cause the nurse practice acts to become less vague as nurse practitioners attempt to limit the number of nurses from becoming qualified to function as nurse practitioners.

52. Council on Health Manpower, *The Physicians' Assistant—A Progress Report* (Chicago: Illinois: American Medical Association, 1971).

53. Richard A. Smith, Gerald R. Bassett, Cornick A. Markarian, Raymond E.

Vath, William L. Freeman, and G. Frederick Dunn, "A Strategy for Health Manpower—Reflections on an Experience Called Medex," *Journal of the American Medical Association*, Vol. 217, No. 10, September 6, 1971, p. 1364.

54. Hepner and Hepner, *The Health Strategy Game*, p. 226.

55. Lave, Lave, and Morton, "The Physicians' Assistant," p. 48. One advantage of this increased amount of leisure time would be the opportunity to upgrade medical skills.

56. Rodney M. Coe and Leonard Fichtenbaum, "Utilization of Physician Assistants: Some Implications for Medical Practice," *Medical Care*, November-December 1972, Vol. 10, No. 6, p. 502. It is possible that the full-time supervision may only be required initially until changes occur in staff attitudes toward the physicians' assistant.

57. Richard Zeckhauser and Michael Eliastam, "The Productivity Potential of the Physician Assistant," *The Journal of Human Resources*, Vol. 9, No. 1, Winter, 1974, p. 114.

58. Ibid.

59. T.G. Grupenhoff and Steven Strickland (Eds.), *Federal Laws: Health, Environment, and Manpower*, Sourcebook Series, Vol. 1 (Washington, D.C.: The Science and Health Communications Group, 1972), p. 4.

60. Grupenhoff and Strickland, *Federal Laws*, p. 9.

61. Ibid., p. 17.

62. Douglas A. Fenderson, "Health Manpower Development and Rural Services," *Journal of the American Medical Association*, September 24, 1973, Vol. 225, No. 13, p. 1629.

63. Carl E. Taylor, Rahmi Dirican, and Durt W. Deuschle, *Health Manpower in Turkey: An International Case Study* (Baltimore, Maryland: The Johns Hopkins Press, 1968), p. 268.

64. John M. Last, "Health Manpower in International Perspective," *The Milbank Memorial Fund Quarterly*, Vol. 48, No. 2, April, 1970, Part I, p. 221.

65. Thomas L. Hall, *Health Manpower in Peru: A Case Study in Planning* (Baltimore, Maryland: The Johns Hopkins Press, 1969), p. 44.

66. F. Harbison and C.A. Myers, *Education, Manpower, and Economic Growth* (New York: McGraw Hill Book Co., 1964).

67. Taylor, Dirican, and Deuschle, *Health Manpower in Turkey*, p. 228.

68. Timothy D. Baker and Mark Perlman, *Health Manpower in a Developing Economy: Taiwan, A Case Study in Planning* (Baltimore, Maryland: The Johns Hopkins Press, 1967), p. 145.

69. Last, "Health Manpower," p. 224.

70. N.R.E. Fendall, *Auxiliaries in Health Care: Programs in Developing Countries* (Baltimore, Maryland: The Johns Hopkins Press, 1972), pp. 34-35.

71. N.R.E. Fendall, "The Auxiliary in Medicine," *Israel Journal of Medical Sciences*, Vol. 4, No. 3, May-June 1968, pp. 616-17.

72. Carl E. Taylor, "Training Health Auxiliaries," paper presented at the

East-West Center for Cultural Technical Inter-Change Conference on Public Health Training and Education in Asian Countries, Honolulu, Hawaii, June 22, 1965, p. 3.

73. Fendall, "The Auxiliary in Medicine," p. 620.

74. Taylor, "Training Health Auxiliaries," pp. 10, 12, and 13.

75. Rosemary Stevens and Joan Vermeulen, *Foreign Trained Physicians and American Medicine*, Bureau of Health Manpower Education (Washington, D.C.: U.S. Government Printing Office, 1972), p. XV.

76. Stevens and Vermeulen, *Foreign Trained Physicians*, p. 1.

77. Ibid., p. 19.

78. Robert J. Weiss, Joel C. Kleinman, Ursula Brandt, and Dan Felsenthal, "The Effect of Importing Physicians—A Return to a Pre-Flexnerian Standard," *New England Journal of Medicine*, Vol. 290, No. 26, June 27, 1974, p. 1455.

79. Weiss, et al., "The Effect of Importing Physicians," p. 1456.

80. Irene Butter and Richard Schaffner, "Foreign Medical Graduates and Equal Access to Medical Care," *Medical Care*, March-April 1971, Vol. 9, No. 2, p. 136.

81. Richard Schaffner and Irene Butter, "Geographic Mobility of Foreign Medical Graduates and the Doctor Shortage: A Longitudinal Analysis," *Inquiry*, Vol. 9, No. 1, March 1972, p. 32.

82. James E. Jonish, "U.S. Physician Manpower and Immigration," *Nebraska Journal of Economics and Business*, Summer, 1971, Vol. 10, No. 3, p. 20.

83. Jonish, "U.S. Physician Manpower and Immigration," p. 16.

84. Harold Luft, *Determinants of the Flow of Physicians to the United States* (Santa Monica, California: Rand Corporation P-4538, December 1970), p. 21.

4 Hospital Costs and Reimbursement

Since 1950 the fraction of income spent by Americans for hospital care has risen steadily. In 1972 the figure reached $33 billion, not including expenditures for construction, research, or the carrying charges for hospital insurance. These latter items accounted for an additional $6 billion in expenditures.[1] Perhaps, another $9 billion went for physicians' and other services rendered within hospitals. Clearly the hospital industry is a major one in the American economy.

Its role in modern health services can hardly be exaggerated. Physical and intellectual center of the medical world, it is the doctors' indispensable workshop, where the three essential elements of scientific medicine—patient care, research, and teaching—are increasingly focused. The hospital is also gradually becoming a community health center, the one institution with the potential for encompassing and integrating the wide range of comprehensive medical services—prevention, treatment, rehabilitation, and after-care.[2]

Hospital care accounts for a much larger portion of national health expenditures than any other category, about 40 percent in 1973. If construction and research costs were added, the figure would reach 47 percent, more than twice as much as the next largest category, physicians' services.[3] If the expenditures for medical services received in the hospital, but allocated to other categories were included, the hospital portion would exceed 60 percent.

In 1872 the ratio of total hospital beds (short-term and long-term) per 1,000 population was less than two. In 1945, because of the World War II expansion in military beds, a peak of 13 per 1,000 was reached. Since that time the number of beds per 1,000 population has fallen irregularly to about 8, representing 1.55 million beds in 7,061 institutions.

Of these some 5,800 with 884,000 beds are nonfederal short-term hospitals, the group with which this chapter is primarily concerned. They account for 93 percent of all admissions, 77 percent of all employees, and 78 percent of total hospital expenditures.[4] However, they contain only about 55 percent of the occupants because most of the other hospitals are long-term institutions providing custodial care with relatively little turnover. Moreover, long-term hospitals are becoming less important, since short-term general hospitals provide care formerly given in mental and tuberculosis institutions, and because of the increasing availability of nursing homes and other parahospital institutions for custodial care.

The most significant trend data, 1950 to 1972, for nonfederal short-term hospitals are presented in Table 4-1. The number of beds per 1,000 population increased 26 percent over the 22 year period. Inpatient admissions per 1,000 rose 33 percent reaching a level of 147.4 in 1972. Both of these rates have shown steady increases throughout the period under consideration. The average length of stay declined from 1950 to 1960 and stabilized thereafter. However, the inpatient population in absolute numbers (average daily census) has continued to rise and reached 664,000 in 1972.

Outpatient care is an increasingly important hospital activity. Unfortunately, complete data are not available for these important services. However, incomplete statistics indicate a steep rise, especially in emergency room and private diagnostic services. From 1957 to 1972 outpatient visits increased from 66 million to 167 million, an increase of over 150 percent. This was nearly three times as rapid as the rate of increase in inpatient admissions.

Full-time personnel (or their equivalents in part-time workers) rose 109 percent to 2.1 million in 1972. The personnel-patient ratio rose 74 percent to a 1972 high of 3.1 employees per patient. In spite of the rise in personnel and higher wages and salaries, payroll as a percent of total expenses changed very little over the entire period indicating that other expenses rose as fast as payrolls.

Total expense per patient day, the hospitals' average per diem cost, rose steadily from 1950 to 1972, a total of 574 percent to a high of $105.21. The very slight decline in length of stay was not nearly enough to offset such cost increases, and the average expense per patient stay advanced 553 percent to $831.

An important indicator of changing hospital operations, not shown in Table 4-1, is the rising number of institutions with specialized technical facilities. Virtually all nonfederal short-term hospitals have a clinical laboratory and diagnostic x-ray equipment compared with 76 and 86 percent respectively in 1946. The proportion of these hospitals with cardiac intensive care units rose from 29 percent in 1967 to 42 percent in 1972. The percentage of hospitals with registered pharmacists increased from 63 percent in 1967 to 87 percent in 1972.[5]

Types of Hospitals

There are a number of different kinds of hospitals. As indicated earlier, this chapter does not consider long-term hospitals. Moreover, federal hospitals will be excluded from analyses because they are not generally accessible to the public. Even within the designation "nonfederal short-term," there are numerous classifications. The 1970 distribution according to ownership and relative size is as follows:[6]

	Percentage		
	Hospitals	Beds	Assets
Voluntary	58.0	69.8	76.9
Proprietary	13.1	6.2	3.3
State and local government	28.9	24.0	19.8
Total, nonfederal short-term	100.0	100.0	100.0

The state and local hospitals are owned and operated by municipalities, counties, or states. In heavily populated or urbanized areas they tend to serve mainly the indigent and low-income patients. Charges have generally been related to income. However, in some localities, the county hospital is the only hospital within a broad geographic area and serves the entire population.

The proprietary hospital is a business enterprise, usually owned and operated by groups of doctors in connection with their medical practice, but sometimes as a separate business activity. Such hospitals may also be owned by other private investors.[7]

The proprietary hospitals are guided by profit considerations in determining the range of services offered and the prices to be charged for these services. Thus, they behave similarly to profit-making enterprises in other industries. Normally these hospitals limit their care to full-pay patients, avoiding the indigent. However, with the government paying full "reasonable costs" under Medicare, on behalf of the aged poor, proprietaries have increased the proportion of low-income elderly patients.

The voluntary hospital is neither a public enterprise nor is it a profit-making institution. Ownership is vague, as the original capital is usually raised through community drives or philanthropy.[8] A substantial number are controlled by Catholic and other religious groups. The voluntary hospital is legally operated by a board of trustees, usually composed of prominent community figures.

Some of the nonprofit aspects of the voluntary hospital are disappearing. The charity patient is more likely to go elsewhere, and because of Medicaid and Medicare there are fewer charity patients. Increasingly the voluntary hospital expects to be paid at least at the level of costs for services rendered. Both proprietary and voluntary hospitals hope to produce a "profit" in the sense that current operating revenues will exceed costs. The difference between them lies in what is done with the surplus. None of the voluntaries' surplus can be distributed to the "owners"; it is all ultimately reinvested in expansion, renovation, or improvement.

As indicated earlier, the voluntary hospital is predominant in the American hospital system. Therefore, most of the subsequent analysis of hospital costs and reimbursement focuses on them.

Table 4-1
United States Nonfederal Short-term Hospitals: Selected Data, 1950-72

	1950	1960	1965	1972	Percent Increase		
					1950-72	1960-65	1965-72
Total civilian resident population (in thousands)	150,790	178,153	191,874	208,837	38.5	7.7	8.8
Number of hospitals	5,031	5,407	5,736	5,843	16.1	6.1	1.9
Number of beds (in thousands)	505	639	741	884	75.0	16.0	19.3
Beds per 1,000 population	3.35	3.59	3.86	4.23	26.3	7.5	9.6
Admission (in thousands)	16,663	22,970	26,943	30,777	84.7	15.2	14.2
Admissions per 1,000 population	110.5	128.9	137.9	147.4	33.4	7.0	6.9
Average daily census (in thousands)	372	477	563	644	78.5	18.0	17.9
Patient days per 1,000 population	900	977	1,071	1,174	30.4	9.6	9.3
Occupancy (percent)	73.7	74.7	76.0	75.2	2.0	1.7	-1.1
Average length of stay (days)	8.1	7.6	7.8	7.9	-2.5	2.6	1.3
Total expenses (in millions)	$ 2,120	$ 5,617	$ 9,147	$25,549	1105.1	62.8	179.3
Total expenses per patient day	$ 15.62	$ 32.23	$ 44.48	$105.21	573.6	38.0	136.5

Expense per patient stay	$127.26	$244.53	$346.94	$831.16	553.1	41.9	139.9
Expense per patient stay in 1972 dollars	$221.31	$345.52	$460.04	$831.16	275.6	33.1	80.7
Expense per capita of population	$ 14.06	$ 31.53	$ 47.67	$122.34	770.2	51.2	156.6
Expense per capita of population in 1972 dollars	$ 24.45	$ 44.55	$ 63.21	$122.34	400.4	41.9	93.5
Full-time personnel (in thousands)*	662	1,080	1,386	2,056	210.6	28.3	48.3
Full-time personnel per 100 patients*	178	226	246	310	74.2	8.8	26.0
Payroll expenses (in millions)	$ 1,203	$ 3,499	$ 5,644	$14,519	1106.9	61.3	157.2
Payroll expenses per patient day	$ 8.86	$ 20.08	$ 27.44	$ 59.79	574.8	36.7	117.9
Payroll expenses per patient day in 1972 dollars	$ 15.41	$ 28.37	$ 36.39	$ 59.79	288.0	28.3	64.3
Average payroll expense per employee	$ 1,817	$ 3,239	$ 4,072	$ 7,062	288.7	25.7	73.4
Payroll expense as percent of total expense	56.7	62.3	61.7	56.8	0.2	-1.0	-7.9
Total assets (in millions)	$ 4,349	$10,858	$16,364	$33,629	673.3	50.7	105.5

*Includes part-time equivalents, except in 1950.

Source: Data for 1950-65 from American Hospital Association, *Hospitals*, Guide Issue, Vol. 40, August 1, 1966, pp. 427-28; and American Hospital Association, *Hospital Statistics, 1972* (Chicago, Illinois: American Hospital Association, 1973), pp. 19-21.

The doctor's relationship to the hospital has become increasingly complex as its role in his professional life has become more important. Although the degree of his association varies with the type of practice, probably at least 50 percent of the average physician's income is earned in the hospital. A surgeon or radiologist may earn up to 100 percent of his income there. In any case, while the physician is the key and indispensable figure in the hospital, with wide authority and latitude, he is not part of the administrative or financial structure. Moreover, a united and determined medical staff can take over a hospital effectively and operate it almost independently without any of the financial risks or responsibilities that it otherwise would face.

Returns to Scale in Hospitals

Conceptually, the question of the existence of returns to scale is straight-forward. In the production of hospital services, just as in the production of any good or service, certain resources, or factors of production, are utilized as inputs in order to obtain a given output. Returns to scale are concerned with the relationship that exists between the inputs and the output. Specifically, the question of returns to scale focuses on what happens to the level of output as the quantity of inputs increases. If the inputs are increased in equal proportional amounts, and output grows at a constant rate, then there are constant returns to scale (constant costs); if output grows at an increasing rate, there are increasing returns to scale (decreasing costs); and if output rises at a decreasing rate, there are decreasing returns to scale (increasing costs).

Economies of scale can result from the specialization of factors of production. For example, the division of labor may permit greater specialization resulting in increased productivity. It seems reasonable to expect that division and specialization of nursing services in hospitals would result in economies of scale. These economies may also result from the use of certain indivisible factors of production. To the extent that certain "lumpy" inputs were required in the production of hospital services, economies of scale would result from the use or combination of factors in more efficient proportions concomitant with higher levels of output. A number of facilities might be suggested that seem to be indivisible in this sense. It is probably impossible, for example, to construct one-half of a pathology laboratory.[9]

Diseconomies of scale, if they exist at all, are usually associated with the inefficiencies of very large-scale management. For example, if a hospital becomes sufficiently large, the burden of administration may become so great that average costs would rise.

Economics textbooks have generally depicted long-run average cost curves as being U-shaped (Figure 4-1). The reason for this is that at lower levels of output economies of scale are important, but at higher levels of output all of these

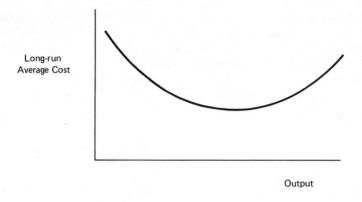

Long-run
Average Cost

Output

Figure 4-1. Long-run Average-cost Curve

economies are fully exploited and the diseconomies of exceedingly large scale may have a major influence on costs. The concept of an optimal size follows from the balancing of these forces. If average cost first falls and then rises as the level of output increases, the optimal size is that which coincides with a minimum average cost.

The existence of economies of scale in the production of hospital services is significant from a policy viewpoint. First, the prevalence of nonprofit enterprises in this industry implies that certain incentives for efficiency that are present in profit-making enterprises are missing or inoperative in the hospital industry. Moreover, forces external to the market influence the construction of new facilities and the expansion of existing facilities. Rational planning requires some indication of the relationship between hospital size and hospital costs.[10] Thus, planning agencies need to know whether or not there is an optimal size for different types of hospitals.

Two empirical methods have been utilized to determine the relationship between cost and output in a firm or group of firms. One approach has been to select a particular firm and study its costs and output over a period. This is known as the time-series method. The other approach, which is used in virtually all hospital cost studies, is to select a particular time period and observe the relationship between cost and output for a large number of firms. In either case, cost analysis is often complicated by variations in product quality and by inability to segregate costs by product for multiproduct firms. Both of these complications are particularly important in an analysis of hospital costs.

Variations in the quality of a particular hospital service undoubtedly exist among hospitals and they probably exist within a single hospital as well. For example, two different hospitals may have facilities for open-heart surgery, but there can be major differences in the quality of care and treatment. Usually higher quality is associated with higher costs of production and, conceptually, cost analysis requires standardization for quality variations.[a] Unfortunately, it is extremely difficult to quantify this particular dimension of quality and its influence on costs cannot be estimated directly.

A further complication for hospital cost analysis results because the output statistics do not reflect differences in the kinds of services provided in different hospitals. Hospitals are essentially multiproduct firms and total costs are not generally segregated for the different products produced. Thus, for example, two hospitals that produce the same range of services may have different average costs because they produce different proportions of these services or a different range of services associated with a dissimilar case mix.

Determination of the optimum allocation of hospital resources involves consideration of both the costs incurred by hospitals themselves and the costs associated with hospitalization that are borne by staff, patients, and visitors. Perhaps the most obvious external cost is travel cost, measured in terms of both dollar outlay and the psychological cost of time consumed.[11]

In any given community, average travel cost per patient day will depend upon a variety of factors such as the location of hospitals, the distribution and characteristics of the population, and the pattern of travel routes. In general, however, one can assume that if the sizes of hospitals were increased (with constant utilization rates), their geographic service areas would expand and, consequently, average travel cost (for both doctors and patients) would rise.[b] In Figure 4-2, line AA relates the average cost per patient day incurred by the hospital to the size of the institution, line BB represents average travel cost, and line CC indicates their sum. Note that the optimum size of a hospital is reduced (from OS_1 to OS_2) when travel cost is considered. While travel cost obviously affects the optimal size and location of hospitals, only the costs actually incurred by hospitals, and reflected in their accounts, have been considered by economists who have done empirical work relating hospital size to cost.

The Measure of Hospital Size

The most obvious measure of hospital size is bed capacity. This measure is used by Herbert E. Klarman, Judith R. and Lester B. Lave, Long, Mann, and Donald Yett, and Kong-Kung Ro and Carl Stevens, in their studies of hospital costs.[12] However, this is not an adequate standard, if size is defined as the average number of patients that can be cared for in an optimal manner. Since hospital

[a]This is the case especially with respect to cardiac surgery. One factor determining the level of quality is whether or not enough operations are done to maintain a high level of skill among the members of the team.

[b]As pointed out by W. John Carr and Paul J. Feldstein, in addition to travel cost, account should be taken of possible increases in morbidity and mortality arising directly from the time it takes to get to hospitals.

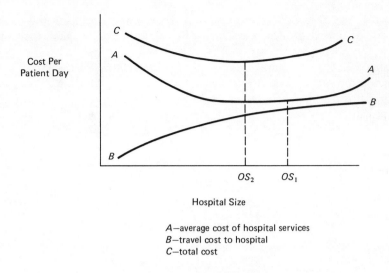

Cost Per
Patient Day

Hospital Size

A—average cost of hospital services
B—travel cost to hospital
C—total cost

Figure 4-2. Relationship Between Hospital Size and Cost

admissions (and discharges) occur randomly over time, a hospital administrator must operate his institution, on the average, at a level of occupancy somewhat lower than minimum capacity in order to provide enough space for unforeseen variations in demand.

One solution to this problem is to use an adjusted bed size measure, which may be determined by subtracting the average number of unoccupied beds from reported bed capacity figures. However, this measure can also present difficulties because of variations in the criteria that hospitals use in determining what shall be counted as bed capacity.[13]

These problems are avoided if average daily census is used as a measure of size. However, sometimes measurement errors may occur although these are generally small relative to variations in average daily census.

The Measure of Output

Almost all studies comparing hospital costs use adult and pediatric patient days as the measure of output. However, as indicated previously, hospitals differ in the number and kind of services that they offer; in general the larger the hospital, the greater the variety of services provided. Many small hospitals, rather than offering a particular service at low volume and consequent high unit cost, will have an agreement with large hospitals in nearby cities to provide this type of service. Such arrangements may reflect insufficient demand in the vicinity of the smaller hospital for either specialized equipment such as Cobalt units or specialist physicians such as neurosurgeons. Thus, merely using patient days as a measure of output involves a systematic bias against larger hospitals that offer many more kinds of services.[14]

Donald E. Saathoff and Richard A. Kurtz have approached this problem by devising a measure of weighted service output that is more inclusive than adult and pediatric days.[15] Their unit of service is

$$S = D + 2A + 0.3\,X + 0.1\,L + 0.2\,O$$

where

$$D = \text{adult and pediatric days}$$

$$S = \text{adjusted measure of output}$$

$$A = \text{surgical and obstetrical admissions}$$

$$X = \text{x-ray diagnostic procedures}$$

$$L = \text{laboratory tests and tissue exams}$$

$$O = \text{outpatient department visits}$$

The weight coefficients used by Saathoff and Kurtz for items D, A, X, L, and O are based on time and motion study.

Harold A. Cohen has developed a measure of output based on cost instead of time and effort per se. His approach to the measure of service output is thus similar to that of Saathoff and Kurtz inasmuch as an adult and pediatric patient day receives a weight of one and the unit cost (in dollars rather than time) of other services is divided by the unit cost of an inpatient day. This, then, gives a measure of output:[16]

$$S^k = W_i Q_i^k$$

$$S^k = \text{service output in the } k\text{th hospital}$$

$$W_i = \text{weight of the } i\text{th service (relative cost)}$$

$$Q_i^k = \text{quantity of } i\text{th service in } k\text{th hospital}$$

Cohen's weighted output measure is an interesting alternative to the measure of output by the number of cases; it solves another problem of empirical analysis, that of controlling for the number of available services and the case-mix variation. The weighted measure must be expanded, however, to include those rare services that are available only in the largest hospitals. Moreover, Cohen's output measure is controversial. It is not obvious that average direct cost is the correct weighting for hospital services; the services that provide a patient with the greatest benefits are not necessarily the most expensive.[17]

Empirical Studies

Table 4-2 summarizes the results of eight fairly recent studies of economies of scale in hospitals.

From this survey of empirical studies on hospital costs, it is apparent that recent research does not permit conclusions about the optimal size of a short-term general hospital. However, the above findings indicate that economies of scale do exist for a substantial range of output beyond the current average size (135 beds) of nonprofit general hospitals in the United States.[18] While there is some evidence that the long-run average cost curve is U-shaped, these studies have not precluded the possibility that the average cost curve is actually L-shaped (first declining then constant average and marginal cost).

It is notable that no detailed analysis of the costs of providing outpatient services has been done. Nor are there any detailed studies relating the costs of outpatient or ambulatory services to the costs of inpatient care. With the volume of outpatient services increasing much faster than inpatient services, this type of research is badly needed. Moreover, further differences in the quality of hospital outputs must also be recognized in the study of returns to scale.

Table 4-2
Findings of Empirical Studies on Hospital Costs

Investigator	Adjustment for Service Capability	Findings
P. Feldstein	None	Declining average cost
Berry	Analysis of groups offering identical services	Declining average cost
Carr and P. Feldstein	Eight measures of service capability and number of services	U-shaped curve; minimum cost at 190 average daily census
Ingbar and Taylor	Four measures of service activity	Inverted U curve; maximum cost at 190 beds
M. Feldstein	Nine case-mix proportions	U-shaped curve but coefficients not statistically significant; minimum cost at 300 beds
Francisco	Index of available services and facilities	Declining average cost
Francisco	Analysis of groups offering identical services	Declining costs for small hospitals*
Cohen	Weighted output measure	Constant costs for larger U-shaped curve; minimum cost at 290-95 beds

*Those offering relatively few services and ranging in size up to about 100 beds.

Source: Thomas R. Hefty, "Returns to Scale in Hospitals: A Critical Review of Recent Research," *Health Services Research*, Vol. 4, No. 4, Winter, 1969, p. 278.

Medicare and Hospital Reimbursement

Public Law 89-97, as passed by Congress in July 1965, amended the basic Social Security Act with the addition of Title XVIII (Medicare).[19] As of July 1, 1966, when the Medicare program went into effect, nearly 18.9 million persons aged 65 and older were enrolled.

The provisions of the Medicare program reflect its erratic course in Congress. While it is considered an insurance scheme, it contains substantial elements of direct subsidy. The benefits provided to those enrolled in the program fall under two categories. Part A of Title XVIII provides for basic hospital insurance and related services, such as posthospital care in an accredited, extended care facility. Under the hospital insurance provisions a beneficiary is covered for up to 90 days as an inpatient in a hospital and 100 days in a nursing home per year. The insurance pays normal charges for semiprivate room or ward plus board, nursing care, and hospital outpatient services. Benefits do not cover (1) care in a private room unless "medically necessary," (2) private duty nursing; (3) services provided in a federal hospital; (4) costs of special services such as telephone or television; and (5) care in foreign hospitals except in emergencies.[20]

The second basic provision of the Medicare Act is for voluntary supplementary medical insurance (SMI) known as Part B coverage. At the start of the program, 17.8 million persons had enrolled for Part B coverage. Those with SMI coverage are entitled to the following services: (1) the care of a physician or surgeon wherever provided; (2) home health care; (3) diagnostic x-rays; (4) laboratory tests; (5) x-ray, radium, and radioactive isotope therapy; (6) ambulance service; and (7) medical appliances.

The normal payment procedure under both Parts A and B takes the form of medical vendor payments. This simply means that the recipient's medical bill is paid directly by the government (or the fiscal intermediary designated by the government) to the supplier of the service. While there are some exceptions to this practice, they do not alter the basic philosophy of providing services directly to recipients rather than the funds necessary to pay for them.

The financing of Medicare reflects the quasi-insurance characteristic of the program. Part A is funded primarily from employer, employee and self-employed contributions under Social Security and the Railroad Retirement Act. Although the act did not require any direct contribution from elderly persons, the program has certain deductible and co-insurance features. In 1974 the recipient was required to pay the first $60 of his hospital bill plus $21 for every day from the 61st to the 90th day of hospitalization. For the next 90 days of hospitalization the patient must pay $42 a day. Supplementary medical insurance coverage under Part B is financed jointly from monthly premiums on recipients (currently the rate is $6.30 per month) and from federal general revenues. As with hospital insurance, the medical supplement has a basic deductible (of $60 per year) plus co-insurance features. A portion of the deductible and co-insurance amounts for the aged, medically indigent under both Parts A and B is financed from Medicaid funds. In all, the program is perhaps best described as heavily subsidized insurance.[21]

Reimbursement

The reasonable cost reimbursement approach for hospitals had been more or less followed by Blue Cross in previous years and was incorporated into the Medicare program. Included in reasonable costs are a number of indirect expenses such as a share of interest on loans, bad debts, the cost of research not paid for by other sources, and the net expense of operating nursing schools. Of course, the usual direct expenses associated with inpatient care are also included. The general principle prevails that the Medicare program is to pay for the actual *cost* of providing care for its beneficiaries. This approach differs from that applicable to private-paying patients, who pay hospitals on the basis of charges (that may bear no specific relationship to the actual costs involved).[22]

It should be recognized that although hospitals are, on the average, in a stronger financial position because of the enactment of Medicare and Medicaid, this is not so in all individual cases.[23] For example, prior to Medicare some large-city private hospitals had relatively few medically indigent aged persons and did not incur losses serving these people due to their pricing structure and good bill collection experience. Frequently, such hospitals undercharged their maternity patients and in the past made up for this by charging more than costs for other patients. Accordingly, these hospitals were adversely affected by the reasonable cost reimbursement of the Medicare program since they no longer made a profit on their patients 65 and over to offset the loss on maternity cases. Of course, these hospitals still had the profit on other nonmaternity patients, under age 65, to offset the maternity losses, but this still resulted in a deterioration of their financial position.[24] Conversely, large-city public hospitals and the nonurban hospitals have been very favorably affected financially under Medicare and Medicaid since most of their aged patients in the pre-Medicare period were indigent.

In the administrative discussions after the enactment of Medicare, it was accepted that the cost of capital facilities, as they are depreciated, should be reimbursable. However, the determination of the level of depreciation created considerable controversy.

Depreciation is the gradual consumption or "using up" of durable assets and the resulting conversion of the assets to expense over the period that the asset is expected to be used. Such expense is customarily based on the original or "historical cost," according to accepted accounting principles.

The hospitals objected to historical cost being the basis for depreciation and insisted that the basis be current replacement costs. The financial implications of the disagreement were substantial. Depreciation is assumed to represent about 6 percent of total reimbursements. Estimates of the difference between reimbursement based on historical, as opposed to replacement, costs range from 50 percent upward.[25]

The hospitals were trying to eliminate a difficult problem through the replacement depreciation proposal—generation of new capital. In the past, hospitals have not generated new capital from operating revenue. Although this practice has been increasing in recent years, only about 35 percent of capital is presently generated internally.

The Social Security Administration maintained that historical cost should be the basis for depreciation, but in recognition of hospital financial problems it has allowed the option of accelerated depreciation in contrast to the straight-line method, which allows an equal amount of depreciation for each year of an asset's life. Moreover, the hospital may use one method of depreciation for one asset or group of assets and another on different assets, in whatever combination is most advantageous.

Most observers of the reimbursement negotiations indicate that the hospital's desire to increase funds for capital formation influenced every major dispute on payments. The most direct claim came in the form of a request for a return on invested capital, not as "profit," for this is explicitly prohibited by the law, but in recognition of "cost" of equity capital.[26] The Social Security Administration indicated that it was sympathetic to the hospital's need for more capital, but did not feel that Medicare was the appropriate vehicle for financing capital formation.

The reimbursement principles developed by the federal government initially consisted of a 2 percent supplement to reasonable costs. At first, this 2 percent factor was stated to be, in part, a recognition of imputed interest on the net capital investment. Later, it was described as being for growth and development and for providing working capital. Finally, it was referred to as an allowance for reasonable costs that are not specifically recognized (because of difficulty in precise measurement).

Effective July 1, 1969, this 2 percent factor was eliminated. This action was taken because the SSA believed that the hospital cost-accounting systems should have become sufficiently sophisticated so that all costs would be adequately recognized.[27]

Reimbursement of institutional providers of medical services on a cost basis has been generally criticized for promoting inefficiency. This criticism has been particularly prevalent in recent years, when hospital costs have risen rapidly. Reimbursement on a cost-plus basis is even less justified since it rewards the inefficient. Accordingly, it has been suggested that hospitals should be given financial rewards when they achieve cost savings (while holding the quality of patient care constant) and conversely, should be financially penalized when their operations are inefficient.

Kong-Kung Ro and Richard Auster have developed an incentive reimbursement approach that is designed to stimulate hospital efficiency. Its three main features are the following: (1) a hospital product is defined as the number and categories of episodes of illness given adequate treatment; (2) the level of efficiency on which the incentive is based is the "standard cost" of each episode of illness—this is the mean cost of that illness (for a given geographic area) plus or minus a number of standard deviations chosen on the basis of the level of efficiency desired; (3) the amount of reimbursement is determined by a weighted average of the actual cost of the case to the hospital and the standard cost as defined above, the weighting factor being chosen to produce the desired degree of incentive.[28]

If coverage under the proposed reimbursement plan were limited to inpatient treatment, hospitals might tend to reduce their costs by substituting outpatient for inpatient care during the patient's recovery and perhaps, also, to admit for inpatient care a larger number of less serious cases in a given diagnostic category. If, however, coverage under the plan proposed by Ro and Auster were extended to outpatient care, so that reimbursement were based on average cost of the *total care* of an illness, efficiency would be increased because both unnecessary admissions and unnecessary days of hospital stay would be discouraged.

With mounting public concern over increasing hospital costs, organizational changes may be forthcoming within which the suggested incentive system could become feasible. Even without any organizational changes, if physicians were made aware of the benefits of efficiency in terms of more funds being made available to hospitals for improvement of facilities and acquisition of new equipment, they might be motivated to support their hospital's efforts to reduce costs. Furthermore, if a doctor consistently used methods of treatment that result in reimbursement to his hospital at less than actual cost, there would be pressure on him to alter his methods.

Ro has strongly argued in favor of marginal cost pricing to increase hospital efficiency; that is, to charge patients in proportion to the charges incurred on their behalf. For example, he advocates giving the public a choice between off-peak and peak-period admissions, with patients receiving a discount in off-peak periods and paying an additional fee for the cost of rush services in peak periods. Incremental pricing, if applied to both hospital charges and the pay scale of hospital personnel, would provide incentive for patients to enter the hospital and for hospital personnel to work on weekends. An incremental pricing system that reflects differences in the value rendered individual patients is already accepted as standard practice with the regulated monopolies.[29]

The most vigorous critic of marginal cost pricing is Sylvester E. Berki:

It is notable that neither Ro nor Weisbrod, the two champions of marginal cost pricing, devote any analytic effort to the interaction between patient and physician preferences; the stochastic nature of demand, . . . the interdependence between ambulatory and inpatient utilization, . . . the incompatibility between price competition and oligopolistic nonprofit industry; the relevance of price competition between tax-paying and some tax-exempt organizations ... to mention a few of those problems which all must be assumed away if ... incremental pricing is to have any validity at all.[30]

Hospital Costs

As the statistics presented in Chapter 1 indicate, hospital costs have been increasing much more rapidly than any other component of the medical care price index. This section explores some of the reasons for the very rapid rise in the price of hospital services and the burden of these costs on consumers.

Because of payments by the government and by insurance companies, changes in the average cost per patient day do not measure the movement of the *net* cost to patients of a day of hospital care.[31] Although the gross cost is the appropriate way to assess hospital inflation, the net costs to patients is sometimes the more relevant statistic for understanding the burden of hospital expenses on individuals. There are three different ways in which net cost may be approximated; each has its own use. (See Table 4-3.)

The cost net of payments by both insurance and government (Net Cost 1) measures the average financial impact on patients of a stay in the hospital. It also indicates the average price that consumers must pay for hospital care. However, since most families do not receive government assistance in paying hospital bills, it is important to study the cost net of insurance but not net of government payments (Net Cost 2). The third definition of net cost—net of payment by government but not net of insurance payments—measures the average cost of purchasing hospital care, whether paid directly or prepaid through insurance (Net Cost 3).

The statistics show that, when deductions are made for payments by insurance companies and government, the cost of an average hospital day has risen only 37 percent since 1950 (Net Cost 1) from $7.59 in 1950 to $10.42 in 1972. If we do not include hospital care paid for by the government (Net Cost 2), the increase is still only 118 percent since 1950. Finally, the figures show that even the total personal cost of care, including insurance benefits (Net Cost 3), rose much more slowly than the average cost per patient day.

Since Net Cost 1 and 2 are measures of the prices that influence patients' demands for hospital care at the time they decide to purchase it, one should compare their increase with that of all consumer prices. Table 4-4 expresses the average cost per patient day and net cost estimates in constant 1957-59 dollars.

The deflated Net Cost 1 shows an unexpected trend—a *decline* of more than 20 percent since 1950. This means that because of the growth of third party payments, the "average" patient at the time of his illness had to forego less of other goods and services in 1972 to buy a day of hospital care than he did in 1950. Under the circumstances it is not surprising that patients' demands for

Table 4-3
Net Cost of Hospital Care

	1950	1955	1960	1966	1968	1972
Proportion of population with private health insurance	50.8	64.7	73.0	81.6	85.8	87.0
Percentage of hospital costs paid by insurance	25.7	39.8	50.0	50.2	44.2	35.9
Percentage of hospital costs paid by government	25.7	23.2	21.4	25.5	40.0	53.7
Average cost per patient day	15.62	23.12	32.23	48.15	61.38	105.21
Net cost 1[a]	7.59	8.58	9.19	11.70	9.70	10.42
Net cost 2[b]	10.22	11.14	11.70	15.70	16.14	22.30
Net cost 3[c]	11.61	17.76	25.33	35.87	36.83	49.24

[a]Net cost 1 = $ACPPD \times \dfrac{\text{Direct Consumer Expenditure}}{\text{Total Expenditure}}$

[b]Net cost 2 = $ACPPD \times \dfrac{\text{Direct Consumer Expenditure}}{\text{Total Private Expenditure}}$

[c]Net cost 3 = $ACPPD \times \dfrac{\text{Total Private Expenditure}}{\text{Total Expenditure}}$

Source: Barbara S. Cooper, Nancy L. Worthington, and Paula A. Piro, "National Health Expenditures, 1929-1973," *Social Security Bulletin*, February 1974, Vol. 37, No. 2, pp. 7-10; Health Insurance Institute, *Source Book of Health Insurance Data, 1973-1974* (New York: Health Insurance Institute, 1974), pp. 19-21; and American Hospital Association, *Hospital Statistics, 1972* (Chicago, Illinois: American Hospital Association, 1973), pp. 19-21.

Table 4-4
Net Cost of Hospital Care Relative to the Consumer Price Index

	1950	1955	1960	1966	1968	1972
Deflated average cost per patient day	$18.64	$24.78	$31.26	$42.57	$50.64	$70.91
Deflated net cost 1	9.06	9.20	8.91	10.34	7.60	7.02
Deflated net cost 2	12.20	11.94	11.35	13.88	12.64	15.03
Deflated net cost 3	13.85	19.04	24.57	31.72	28.84	33.19

Source: Table 4-3 and Consumer Price Indices 1950-72.

more and better hospital services have increased. Even for patients who do not receive government help in paying for hospital care, the real net cost (i.e., deflated Net Cost 2) has risen less than 25 percent in the entire period from 1950 to 1972.

In a major study covering the rise in hospital costs from 1950 to 1968, Martin

S. Feldstein found that increased demand was the primary reason for the unusually rapid rate of cost increase.[32] Rising income and more comprehensive insurance coverage, both public and private, have increased patients' willingness to pay for more and better hospital care. Higher demand has likely induced a change in the technology of hospital care to a better but more costly product. Moreover, increasing demand for hospital care has caused an increase in the demand for hospital personnel, contributing to the relatively rapid rise in hospital wage rates. Minimum wage legislation and the unionization of hospital personnel are also important factors in the significant increase in hospital wages.

The increase in wage rates has accounted for about half of the higher cost per patient day from 1955 to 1968. Although there has been no change in the occupational mix of hospital employees toward more skilled workers, the earnings of hospital employees have increased substantially more than the economy-wide wage level for the reasons indicated above. By 1969 hospital employees often had higher earnings than other workers in the same job categories. Moreover, the rates of wage increase have been as high for professional nursing and technical staff as for the less skilled employees.

As indicated above, one important factor tending to increase the demand for hospital care is health insurance.

The effect of prepaying health care through insurance, is to encourage hospitals to produce a more expensive product than consumers actually wish to purchase at the time of illness. The insured patient's demand for care reflects the net price, the hospitals' charge net of insurance benefits. He is therefore willing to purchase much more expensive care than he would if he were not insured. This induced demand for expensive care gives a "false signal" to hospitals about the type of care the public wants. Unfortunately, the production of high-cost hospital care is a self-reinforcing process; the risk of very expensive hospital care stimulates patients to prepay hospital bills through relatively comprehensive insurance, while the growth of such insurance makes hospital care more expensive.[33]

Using state data on hospital costs for the period from 1958 to 1967, Martin S. Feldstein found that more than half of the rise in costs over that period was attributable to increases in private insurance coverage[34]—a factor that, as indicated above, would tend to stimulate demand.

David Salkever's results also tend to confirm the demand-pull hypothesis of hospital cost inflation. Although Salkever's model of hospital inflation allowed for both demand and factor-supply variables, he found that approximately two-thirds of the increase in New York hospital costs over the period 1961-67 was attributable to demand factors (primarily Medicare and insurance coverage), while the other third was caused by increases in wages and prices of other goods and services.[35]

Karen Davis, examining inflation in the 1962-66 period, concluded that the Feldstein demand-pull model requires modification to be consistent with the observed divergence between hospital prices and costs.

The model should at least be modified to include a lagged response of cost increases to increases in hospital prices. To the extent that the impetus for cost increases would come from patients' demands for improved services, one would expect increases in costs of food service, more nursing service, and building investment to make patients' surroundings more luxurious. There is little evidence that hospital cost inflation has taken this form. Instead, these types of services have risen more slowly than other types of expenses. However, the slight switch to greater use of larger hospitals, may reveal an increasing demand among patients for higher quality care, either actual or perceived.[36]

In a previous section it was implied that hospital costs would be affected by the type of reimbursement plan. However, studies by M.V. Pauly and D.F. Drake,[37] and by Davis[38] have investigated the impact of reimbursement schemes on hospital costs. Neither study found any relation between hospital costs and the extensiveness of cost reimbursement. The Pauly-Drake study analyzed individual hospital data in Illinois, Indiana, Michigan, and Wisconsin for 1966. It revealed that hospitals in states in which Blue Cross reimbursed on the basis of costs do not have higher costs than hospitals in states in which Blue Cross reimbursed on the basis of charges. Davis used state data on hospital costs for the years, 1965, 1967, and 1968, and investigated the joint effect of Blue Cross cost reimbursement plans. She found that hospital costs do not vary with the extensiveness of cost reimbursement. Salkever also found that Blue Cross coverage did not lead to higher hospital costs than other private insurance coverage—confirming the finding that while overall increases in insurance coverage may lead to hospital-cost increases, reimbursement on the basis of costs does not, in itself, lead to higher prices for hospital services.[39]

Policies to Reduce Hospital Costs

One method to lower the rise in hospital costs would be to change the structure of insurance coverage.

At present, most hospitalization plans provide extensive coverage, frequently without cost to the patient, for brief stays. Limits on covered days or total expenses, however, leave some persons poorly protected against large hospital bills.

In order to close these gaps in coverage without inducing further increases in hospital costs, insurance coverage could be restructured to provide less protection against relatively low hospital bills and more coverage for high ones. Since a number of studies cited above have concluded that insurance coverage is itself responsible for hospital inflation, making greater use of deductible and co-insurance provisions may reverse some of the inflationary trends. A maximum ceiling, however, must be placed on the extent of cost sharing so that each family is assured that out-of-pocket expenses will not exceed some reasonable fraction of income.[40]

A variant of this proposal has been made by Joseph P. Newhouse and Vincent Taylor.[41] They would introduce a new type of insurance known as variable cost insurance. Under this plan the proportion of a subscriber's hospital bill paid by insurance would be inversely proportional to the expense rating of the hospital and directly proportional to the expense class rating of his insurance. Under this plan the consumer would bear the full cost of going to hospitals with higher than average costs, and gain the savings from going to hospitals with lower than average costs. This would not only reduce the escalation in hospital costs, but would provide hospitals a powerful motive to improve their performance.

Another policy that might tend to reduce inflationary pressures is the introduction of low-cost alternatives to inpatient care. These incentives might, for example, encourage the proliferation of health maintenance organizations that would emphasize preventive care. In addition, health insurance policies could encourage alternatives to inpatient care by having, for example, lower co-insurance rates for care obtained outside the hospital.

An econometric study by Davis and L.B. Russell found that a 10 percent reduction in the direct price of outpatient visits over and above existing insurance coverage would induce a substitution of hospital outpatient care for inpatient care resulting in a savings in hospital costs of about $40 per 1,000 persons in the population.[42]

Hospitals or Health Centers: A Dilemma for Developing Countries

One of the most important issues facing developing countries today is the trade-off between providing high quality care for a relatively few people in hospitals or lower quality care for a greater number of persons in health centers.

A health center is defined as a unit that provides a family with all the health services it requires, other than those that can only be rendered in a hospital. Each health center is responsible for a specified geographic area. Ideally, the whole country, urban and rural, should be served by health centers. Health centers play a major role in health education. In the rural areas health centers are the fundamental units providing both preventive and curative medical care. The importance of health centers in a developing country can hardly be overemphasized.

In the developing world, it costs approximately $22,000 to build and $11,000 per year to operate a health center providing adequate medical care for 10,000 persons. Similarly, the cost of a hospital bed in a developing country costs $8,000 to provide and $850 per year to service. Considering only annual operating costs, health center facilities can be provided for 1,000 people at an average cost of $1,100. This would service 1.3 hospital beds, in which roughly 100 patients could be treated during one year.[43]

Which policy makes more sense? Is capital better invested in constructing health centers or in providing an additional quarter of a hospital bed for every thousand people? Should these operating funds be used in making health center services available or in servicing about one and a third additional beds for every thousand people? Strict calculations on the return in human welfare from these alternative forms of expenditure are not possible. However, the lower costs of the health center services certainly indicate that once a certain minimal level of hospital services have been provided, then an emphasis should be placed on constructing the former.

It may be argued that the provision of adequate health center services will increase the demand for hospital beds because more cases will be referred for hospital care. While this is true, the exact relationship between the needs for these two kinds of service is complex, and depends on other factors such as the skill of the health center staff in caring for patients, and the use that can be made of home care.

The comparison between the capital cost of hospital and health center services is even more dramatic when considered on a national scale. For example, assume that a country has a population of 8 million. At a cost of $8,000 a bed, it would cost $65 million to provide one bed per 1,000 persons, but to construct an adequate number of health centers would require a capital outlay of only $18 million.

Sixty-five million dollars is a large sum for a developing country to raise and it is useful to consider what a more realistic amount, say $8 million, would accomplish. This would provide 1,000 beds and increase the average number of beds per 1,000 people by one-eighth of a bed. The same amount of funds would have provided full health center services for half the population on the basis of one center for 10,000 people, or almost the entire population at the rate of one for 20,000 people.

The concept of the health center is closely related to the "referral system." This system is based on the idea that patients are to be treated as close to their homes as possible in the smallest, cheapest, most simply equipped, and most humbly staffed unit that will adequately care for them.[44] Only when a particular unit cannot care for a patient adequately is he to be referred to a unit higher up in the chain, the chain being the health center, the district hospital, the regional hospital, and the national hospital.

Treatment at the periphery of a service is much cheaper than that at the center; this is the great advantage of the referral system. (See Table 4-5.) This table based on Kenyan data indicates how much the cost of treating an illness increases as one if referred from the health center to the national hospital. Even allowing for the longer stays in the regional and national hospitals (because of their greater complexity of cases), the difference in average cost is substantial.

Does the referral system work? Not always; sometimes it fails because few hospitals have health centers close enough to them. Transport difficulties also

Table 4-5

Cost Differences, Health Center and Local, Regional, and National Hospitals, Kenya, 1966

Institution	Average Stay	Average Cost Per Illness	Average Cost Per Day
Health center	– – –	$ 0.56	– – –
District hospital	7 days	$11.80	$1.68
Regional hospital	10 days	$24.00	$2.40
National hospital	22 days	$52.00	$2.40

Source: N.R.E. Fendall, "Planning Health Services in Developing Countries, *Public Health Reports,* Vol. 78, 1963, p. 977.

limit the efficiency of the system and often regional and national hospitals must act as district health facilities. For example, about 80 percent of the patients admitted to the New Mulago Hospital, Uganda's national hospital, come from the neighboring district of Mengo, which contains only 20 percent of Uganda's population.[45] However, even with imperfections the referral system is very important, particularly at its lowest level, in which health centers refer cases to the district hospitals.

Distance is a critical factor in the utilization of health services. For example, studies in East Africa have shown a close correlation between proximity and the use of health services. In Uganda the average number of outpatient visits declines by 50 percent for every two miles that people live from a hospital, every one and a half miles from a dispensary, and every mile from an aide post.[46] Whatever the country, few people will walk more than several miles for outpatient services.

The inhibiting influence of distance is an important concern in distributing health facilities. It has been suggested that health facilities be placed so that medical care is within 10 miles of every person. In most countries, an area of 10 mile radius will contain 5,000 to 50,000 people, numbers that can be cared for by the staff of a health center associated with a district hospital for referral. If the Uganda data apply generally, even with the 10 mile spacing, only a small portion of the people (less than 20 percent) will utilize health facilities.[47] This reaffirms the concept that effective health care systems must reach into the communities and homes since it is there that behavioral changes are most likely to be achieved and because people will not travel substantial distances for health care.

Summary

The quantity of hospital services rendered has increased enormously in the past generation. An increasing proportion of care is provided in the nonfederal short-term hospital. Most of these hospitals are operated on a nonprofit basis.

Empirical studies of economies of scale within hospitals fail to indicate whether the long-run average cost curve is U-shaped or L-shaped. However, it is apparent that the optimal size hospital (from the cost minimization standpoint) would be larger than the bed capacity of most voluntary hospitals.

Most health experts have argued that reimbursement on the basis of costs is inefficient. However, studies of various reimbursement plans have failed to indicate that hospitals which are reimbursed on the basis of costs have higher expense levels than those which are reimbursed on the basis of charges.

The primary cause of rising hospital costs is higher demand for hospital services, which is stimulated by the prevalence of hospital insurance. Rapid increases in wages of hospital personnel constitutes an important secondary factor.

Health centers in developing countries are much more economical, in terms of costs per person treated, than hospitals. This implies that once a minimum level of hospital facilities is provided, the availability of health services to the population can be maximized if emphasis is placed on the construction and operation of health centers.

Notes

1. American Hospital Association, *Hospital Statistics, 1972* (Chicago, Illinois: American Hospital Association, 1973), p. 7.

2. Herman M. Somers and Anne R. Somers, *Medicare and the Hospitals: Issues and Prospects* (Washington, D.C.: The Brookings Institution, 1967), p. 43.

3. Barbara S. Cooper, Nancy L. Worthington, and Paula A. Piro, "National Health Expenditures, 1929-1973," *Social Security Bulletin*, February 1974, Vol. 37, No. 2, p. 7.

4. American Hospital Association, *Hospital Statistics, 1972*, p. 20.

5. Ibid., p. 11.

6. U.S. Department of Health, Education and Welfare, *Medical Care Costs and Prices: Background Book* (Washington, D.C.: U.S. Government Printing Office, 1972), p. 19.

7. Somers and Somers, *Medicare*, p. 49.

8. Ibid.

9. Ralph E. Berry Jr., "Returns to Scale in the Production of Hospital Services," *Health Services Research*, Vol. 2, No. 2, Summer, 1967, p. 125.

10. Ibid.

11. W. John Carr and Paul J. Feldstein, "The Relationship of Cost to Hospital Size," *Inquiry*, Vol. 4, No. 2, June 1967, p. 49.

12. Sylvester E. Berki, *Hospital Economics* (Lexington, Massachusetts: D.C. Heath and Co., 1972), p. 112.

13. Carr and Feldstein, "The Relationship of Cost to Hospital Size," p. 52.

14. Harold A. Cohen, "Variations in Cost Among Hospitals of Different Sizes," *Southern Economic Journal*, Vol. 33, No. 3, January 1967, p. 358.

15. Donald E. Saathoff and Richard A. Kurtz, "Cost Per Day Comparisons Don't Do the Job," *The Modern Hospital*, October, 1962, pp. 14, 16, and 142.

16. Cohen, "Variations in Cost," p. 364.

17. Thomas R. Hefty, "Returns to Scale in Hospitals: A Critical Review of Recent Research," *Health Services Research*, Vol. 4, No. 4, Winter, 1969, p. 276.

18. Hefty, "Returns to Scale," p. 275.

19. Margaret Greenfield, Medicare and Medicaid: *The 1965 and 1967 Social Security Amendments* (Berkeley, California: University of California Institute of Governmental Studies, 1968), p. 1.

20. Bruce Stuart and Lee Bair, *Health Care and Income: The Distributional Impacts of Medicaid and Medicare Nationally and in the State of Michigan* (Michigan: Michigan Department of Social Services, September 1971), Research Paper No. 5, Second Edition, p. 15.

21. Stuart and Bair, *Health Care and Income*, p. 16.

22. Robert J. Myers, *Medicare* (Homewood, Illinois: Richard D. Irwin, 1970), p. 129.

23. See for example, Paul J. Feldstein and Saul Waldman, "The Financial Position of Hospitals in the First Two Years of Medicare," *Inquiry*, Vol. 6, No. 1, March 1969, pp. 19-27.

24. Myers, *Medicare*, p. 130.

25. Somers and Somers, *Medicare*, p. 171.

26. Ibid., p. 178.

27. Myers, *Medicare*, p. 134.

28. Kong-Kung Ro and Richard Auster, "An Output Approach to Incentive Reimbursement for Hospitals," *Health Services Research*, Fall, 1969, p. 178.

29. Kong-Kung Ro, "Incremental Pricing Would Increase Efficiency in Hospitals," *Inquiry*, Vol. 6, No. 1, March 1969, p. 32.

30. Berki, *Hospital Economics*, pp. 180-81.

31. Martin S. Feldstein, *The Rising Cost of Hospital Care* (Washington, D.C.: Information Resources Press, 1971), p. 13.

32. Feldstein, *Rising Cost*, p. 74.

33. Ibid., p. 76.

34. Martin S. Feldstein, "Hospital Cost Inflation: A Study of Nonprofit Price Dynamics," *American Economic Review*, Vol. 61, No. 5, December 1971, p. 870.

35. David Salkever, "A Microeconometric Study of Hospital Cost Inflation," *Journal of Political Economy*, Vol. 80, 1972, pp. 1160-61.

36. Karen Davis and Richard W. Foster, *Community Hospitals: Inflation in the Pre-Medicare Period* (Washington, D.C.: U.S. Government Printing Office,

1972), U.S. Department of Health, Education and Welfare, Social Security Administration, Office of Research and Statistics, Research Report 41, p. 52.

37. M.V. Pauly and D.F. Drake, "Effect of Third Party Methods of Reimbursement on Hospital Performance," in Herbert E. Klarman (Ed.), *Empirical Studies in Health Economics* (Baltimore, Maryland: The Johns Hopkins Press, 1970), pp. 297-314.

38. Karen Davis, "Theories of Hospital Inflation: Some Empirical Evidence," *Journal of Human Resources*, in press.

39. Karen Davis, "Rising Hospital Costs: Possible Causes and Cures," *Bulletin of the New York Academy of Medicine*, Vol. 48, No. 11, December 1972, p. 1367.

40. Martin S. Feldstein, "A New Approach to National Health Insurance," *The Public Interest*, Vol. 23, Spring, 1971, p. 99.

41. Joseph P. Newhouse and Vincent Taylor, "The Subsidy Problem in Hospital Insurance: A Proposal," *Journal of Business*, Vol. 43, No. 4, October 1970, pp. 452-56.

42. Karen Davis and L.B. Russell, "The Substitution of Hospital Outpatient Care for Inpatient Care," *Review of Economics and Statistics*, Vol. 54, No. 2, May 1972, p. 119.

43. Richard Jolly and Maurice King, "The Organization of Health Services," in Maurice King (Ed.), *Medical Care in Developing Countries* (London, England: Oxford University Press, 1966), pp. 2-12.

44. Jolly and King, "The Organization of Health Services," pp. 2-4.

45. P.J.S. Hamilton and A. Anderson, "The Admission of Patients to Mulago Hospital," unpublished, 1965; Uganda General African Census, 1959.

46. Jolly and King, "The Organization of Health Services," pp. 2-7.

47. John Bryant, *Health and the Developing World* (Ithaca, New York: Cornell University Press, 1969), p. 130.

5

The Costs and Benefits of Health Programs

Cost-benefit analysis is a series of mathematical calculations that provide an estimate of the potential value of undertaking a given course of action such as instituting a new program or revising an old one.[1] In cost-benefit analysis, the monetary cost of a program is normally compared with its expected benefits, and usually these benefits are expressed in dollars.

In a cost-benefit analysis of alternative programs, one compares the expected benefits and costs of each to determine which should receive priority funding. Because of the frequent emphasis on the most efficient use of funds when given a choice of possible programs, the value of benefits divided by cost, the benefit-cost ratio, is often useful in making comparisons of alternative programs.[2]

For example, assume that one had to make a choice as to which of the following six programs would be funded:

Program	Benefit/Cost Ratio	Cost of Program
A	12:1	$40,000
B	10:1	60,000
C	9:1	20,000
D	8:1	80,000
E	4:1	10,000
F	2:1	18,000

Assume that total expenditures were limited to $120,000. If cost-benefit ratios were the only criteria used for project selection, projects A, B, and C would be funded and the others would not.

Because public projects often yield benefits accruing in the future, these benefits must be discounted by an appropriate interest rate in order to determine their present value. For example, suppose that one is contemplating the construction of a dam. The dam is expected to yield services for a period of 50 years. Let us assume that the annual dollar benefit of the dam is equal to $200,000 per year. The total expected benefits of the dam are equal to

$$\Sigma B = \frac{\$200,000}{(1+r)} + \frac{200,000}{(1+r)^2} + \frac{200,000}{(1+r)^3} + \frac{200,000}{(1+r)^4} + \ldots + \frac{200,000}{(1+r)^{50}}$$

Similarly, if the construction of the dam would take 5 years at a cost of $3 million per year, the total expected costs would be:

$$\Sigma C = \frac{\$3,000,000}{(1+r)} + \frac{3,000,000}{(1+r)^2} + \ldots + \frac{3,000,000}{(1+r)^5}$$

The total benefits (ΣB) are then divided by the total cost (ΣC) to obtain the benefit-cost ratio.

Thus, the discounting process, which recognizes that a given sum of money to be spent or realized in the future is not worth the same amount as the equivalent dollar value obtained or allocated today, provides a link between present value or cost and expected future benefits or costs.

Some health personnel and program planners object to a major reliance on cost-benefit analysis to evaluate health programs. They feel these projects should be justified on the basis of noneconomic or humanitarian considerations. While this writer agrees in part with this position, it is clear that the economic costs and benefits of health programs are one vitally important type of information that decision makers require in order to formulate appropriate policy and to establish priorities. For as Henry Bixby Hemenway has written:

Public health administration is a business. As such, it is subject to ordinary commercial laws, may be judged by commercial standards, and compared with other lines of economic activity. . . . Cities, counties, states, and nations do not have unlimited funds for their various activities. Judged according to commercial standards the funds at their disposal should be applied where and in proportion as they will produce the greatest returns.[3]

Early Studies

Antecedent to research evaluating the benefits and costs of the elimination of specific diseases or of particular health programs were attempts to estimate the monetary value of human life. The earliest recorded systematic work is probably that of Sir William Petty's *Political Arithmetick* in which he assessed the "capital value per capita: of the English population."[4] He calculated the rate of return obtained by moving the London population outside the city during epidemics of the plague. He also calculated the cost-benefit ratio of this endeavor as well as the benefits received from immigration and migration, and also the economic benefits in terms of lives saved attributed to improvements in medical care.[5]

Petty's analysis was highly sophisticated but so far as one is able to determine, it had little impact on other economists or on formulators of public policy. It remained for Edward Chadwick to unite the concept of human capital with health and disease factors into an effective set of public policy recommendations. Chadwick's Report on the Sanitary Condition of the Working

Population of Great Britain (1842) represented four years of superb field investigation and a much longer period of concern for the social costs of the Industrial Revolution in England.[6] This study was the first attempt to link disease and health factors directly to economic, social, and demographic variables. His findings contained four major conclusions:

1. The existence of a strong correlation between environmental variables such as poor sanitation and drainage, inadequate water supply and overcrowded housing and disease, high mortality rates and low life expectancy.
2. The heavy economic cost of illness to society as measured by the loss in productive labor. His estimates of the value (human capital) for individuals were based on the costs of raising a child until he reached the age at which he became productive.[7]
3. The existence of social costs (crime, low moral standards) that were associated with poverty and poor housing.
4. The lack of existing public policy and administration to deal effectively with these three important issues.

Chadwick's report and his subsequent writings and lobbying led ultimately (in 1848) to the passage of the Public Health Act, a landmark in the history of public health movements.

William Farr, in a paper published in 1853, calculated the "capitalized value of man's earning capacity," not by using the costs of rearing children or of producing a member of the labor force, but on the basis of the future income stream of workers (English agricultural laborers) of different ages discounted to the present.[8] Farr also subtracted consumption expenditures from his calculation of earning capacity in order to obtain a net figure, a procedure that was neglected until very recently.

Toward the end of the nineteenth century, Max von Pettenkofer stated that the monetary value of health to a city (Munich) consisted of the average loss of wages while sick and the costs of medical care (leaving aside the losses due to premature death).[9] However, he argued that value of life and health, of increased vitality and longer life cannot be expressed in money terms. Pettenkofer also discussed the public and private benefits to be gained from the implementation of public health programs, and his work can be thought of as a primitive form of cost-benefit analysis.[10]

Early work in the United States was undertaken by the economist Irving Fisher under the auspices of the National Conservation Commission. Fisher's goal was a "money appraisal of preventable wastes," that is, losses sustained due to preventable deaths, loss of working time by sick members of the labor force, and the cost of medical treatment. The monetary calculations were based on Farr's earlier estimates, with adjustments made to allow for the differences between English and American wage rates. He concluded that "The actual economic saving annually possible in this country by preventing needless deaths, needless fatigue, is certainly far greater than $1.5 billion and may be 3 or more times as great."[11]

Twenty years later another classic in the field was published by L.I. Dublin and A.J. Lotka. In their monograph, *The Money Value of a Man*, they focused on how a man might protect his family against economic loss should he die prematurely, and their book constituted an examination of "the value of a man to persons who have a direct interest in his earnings," rather than his value to society per se. They, too, based their estimates on the value of future earning power (discounted at 2.5 percent) less consumption and maintenance during childhood, the working years, and old age.

Cost-benefit Methodology

In cost-benefit analysis as applied to the health field the total cost of the disease serves as the measure of benefits derived from preventing or eradicating the disease.[12] Costs comprise three elements: (1) loss of production; (2) expenditures for medical care; and (3) the pain, discomfort, and suffering that accompany a disease. Because economists concentrate on measuring the first two elements, the third is often neglected for lack of data and an appropriate methodology.

Expenditures for medical care to treat a disease (or injury) are not the total costs of that disease. The economic costs of illness comprise at least two components: direct costs and indirect costs. Direct costs are the expenditures for health services attributable to the disease, such as costs for inpatient care, physicians' fees, and drugs. These expenditures reflect the use of resources. Indirect costs are associated with the loss of output attributable to the disease owing to premature death or disability.

Thus, the total (direct plus indirect) costs of a disease serve as a measure of benefits derived from a program that would achieve eradication or control of disease. In a cost-benefit calculation the comparison is between contemplated additional expenditures for health services and the anticipated reduction in existing costs. This is the essential conceptual framework.

Utilizing information on the direct and indirect costs of illness in 1963, Dorothy P. Rice computed the total costs of illness for diseases of the circulatory system. (See Table 5-1.) Notice that indirect costs (primarily premature mortality) constitute nearly nine-tenths of total cost.

The total economic costs of illness, disability, and death for all diseases was estimated by Rice to be $58 billion in 1963. She estimated that the gross national product in 1963 would have been 3.6 percent higher if the total population had been free of illness.[13]

During 1963, $23.8 billion was lost to the economy due to premature or

Table 5-1
Estimated Economic Cost for Diseases of the Circulatory System, 1963

Type of Cost	(Millions)	Percent
Total	20,948.3	100.0
Direct costs	2,267.3	10.8
Hospital care	1,272.7	
Nursing home care	207.1	
Physicians' services	714.2	
Nursing care[a]	73.3	
Indirect costs		89.2
Morbidity losses–1963		
Institutional population	328.9	
Noninstitutional population	2,590.7	
Mortality losses–1963 and future years, discounted at 4 percent	15,761.4	

[a]Includes the services of private duty professional nurses in the hospital and home, private duty practical nurses, and visiting nurses.

Source: Dorothy P. Rice, *Estimating the Cost of Illness* (Washington, D.C.: U.S. Government Printing Office, May 1966), U.S. Department of Health, Education, and Welfare, Public Health Service, Publication No. 947-6, pp. 8, 20, 32, and 42.

preretirement death, illness, and disability from all diseases. Mortality losses accounted for 11.5 percent of the total, and the remaining 88.5 percent were morbidity losses.

To calculate the economic loss from premature mortality, the estimated value of all deaths is the product of the number of deaths and the expected value of an individual's future earnings.[14] This method of calculation must consider the changing pattern of earnings at successive ages, varying labor force participation rates, work life expectancy for different age and sex groups, and the appropriate discount rate to convert a stream of costs or benefits into its present worth.

In order to estimate rigorously the present value of future losses resulting from morbidity, longitudinal data are required on the patterns of illness by diagnosis. If a particular illness strikes an individual in the early years of his working life, how will this affect his productivity in future years? Some illnesses may totally incapacitate him for part of his life, still others may result in a lifetime of partial disability. Although a person cannot die twice, he can be ill or disabled from the same disease more than once.[15] If one can obtain longitudinal data relating to morbidity patterns by diagnosis the analyst can assess the total economic impact of morbidity from specific illnesses. When longitudinal data are not available (which is generally the case) estimates are simply made by multiplying the individual's annual earnings by the fraction of the year he is not available for productive work. This procedure, of course, ignores losses in future earning power associated with the illness.

Methodological Issues

The Discount Rate

As indicated previously, a given amount of money has different values when it is realized or spent at different times. The process of discounting converts a stream of benefits into its present value: The higher the rate of discount the lower the present value of a future income stream. Discounting is particularly important when a long time span is involved, as in a public program where some benefits accrue 30 to 50 years after the outlay.

Fairly small variations in the discount rate can often lead to major differences in the benefit-cost ratio. To illustrate this, consider an activity costing $100 a year. Assume that by the end of the year $100 has been spent, and the resultant benefit is equivalent to $110. Without doing any discounting (zero percent) the net benefit in dollars is $110 - 100$ or 10.

If a discount rate of 5 percent were employed, the net program benefit would be approximately $5, $[(\frac{110}{1.05}) - 100]$, and were a 10 percent discount rate chosen, the net program benefit would be zero, $[\frac{\$110}{1.10} - 100]$.

What rate of discount should be employed? The discount rate should represent the value of the funds if available for other uses (opportunity cost). Of course, the funds could be used in a number of different sectors. If one considers the government sector, the money is worth what the government pays to borrow it, that is, the interest rate on long-term government bonds. Others have argued that the discount rate should measure the cost of using private capital; as such, the proper rate should be that charged by commercial banks for business loans. However, this might not always be appropriate; the discount rate is meant to balance the productivity of an investment and the reluctance of society to sacrifice current for future consumption. Thus, the individual's market calculations and collective calculations need not coincide.[16] It may be necessary to employ a rate that synthesizes the social rate of discount and opportunity cost (income foregone) in the private sector.[17]

Burton Weisbrod sees the selection of a discount rate as tantamount to expressing a value judgment on the relative importance of successive generations. Accordingly he prefers to present two rates—4 percent and 10 percent. He does not explicitly choose between them and presents his calculations regarding the cost of illness on the basis of both rates. Herbert E. Klarman also believes that it is appropriate to utilize a range of rates when calculating the benefits of programs, but in his study of syphilis he uses a discount rate of 4 percent.[18] However, others employ a "market" rate of interest.[19]

The federal government is now struggling with the problem of setting a standard interest rate for use by all federal agencies. This is a difficult task partly because of the political factors involved. For example, it has been noted that every water project would be dropped if even the low rate of government borrowing were used as a criterion; this action would never be accepted by either the legislative or executive branches because of political implications.[20] Moreover, the proponents of highway construction have succeeded in getting legislation passed that requires the Department of Transportation to use very low interest rates in its calculations.[21]

Net Effective Discount Rate

When utilizing a discount rate for purposes of calculating output loss or expected benefits, it is usually assumed that the general price level will remain constant. However, to the extent that changes occur in the prices of health services relative to all prices this should be taken into consideration by computing the net effective discount rate. For example, experience in the recent past indicates that prices charged by physicians are rising faster than the Consumer Price Index. If the discount rate is 4 percent and one assumes that medical care prices will rise 1.25 percent more rapidly than all prices, one obtains the equivalent of an effective net discount rate of 2.72 percent $(1.04 \div 1.0125 = 1.0272)$.[22]

Similar reasoning applies to changes in productivity. If productivity is expected to rise at the rate of 1.75 percent a year, the net effective discount rate is equal to $(1.04 \div 1.0175)$ or 1.0221.

Presence of Multiple Diseases

The existence of several conditions presents difficulties in measuring the economic aspects of each contributing disease or condition. When a person is suffering from more than one disease at the same time, his costs of medical care and production losses cannot be clearly identified with a single disease. The presence of multiple diseases, results in an overstatement of the cost of any one disease when the economic costs are measured separately. The extent of overstatement is affected by the degree of interdependence in the origin of the diseases. Economists generally agree that the total indirect costs of individual diseases cannot be added together to estimate the total costs of disease to society. Methods for measuring the effect of the presence of an additional disease on medical care expenditures have not yet been developed.

Calculation of Output Loss

The appropriate measure of output loss for individuals is year-round, full-time earnings, which includes wages and salaries before tax deductions. The correct measure of expected earnings is the arithmetic average or mean (not the median, which is frequently employed because it is available in various census publications). Adjustments should be made to recognize wage supplements such as employer contributions for social insurance, private pensions and welfare funds.

One could argue that the appropriate measure of output loss is not earnings but output per worker. However, this implies that labor is the only factor of production and ignores the contribution of such factors as land, capital, or entrepreneurship. Yet, in a severe epidemic in which much capital equipment is idle output per worker may be the more appropriate measure of output loss.

Rate of Employment

Not everyone would have been in the labor force or employed even in the absence of morbidity or premature mortality. Some persons are too old or too young to be in the work force while others are unwilling or unable to find jobs. The estimates of losses in output due to death or illness assume that persons stricken would have the same employment experience as others in the same age and sex categories. Labor force participation rates are applied and further adjustments are made for the number who would have been employed under conditions of high employment (generally defined as 4 percent unemployment). For example, assume that the average earnings of males 25 to 34 is $8,000 with a labor force participation rate of 97 percent and an unemployment rate of 4 percent. Then the expected earnings of a 25 to 34 year old male is $8,000 × 0.93 (0.97 − 0.04) or $7,440. However, notice should be taken of the somewhat unfavorable employment prospects of rehabilitated persons in this country.[23] Moreover, it is also likely that differences in employment potential exist between a group in whom a disease has been prevented and one in whom the disease occurs and is cured.

Allowance for Consumption

Diversity of opinion prevails regarding the treatment of consumption. Economists agree that insurance companies and families should deduct consumption in their calculations of the economic value of the bread winner.[24] However, both Rashi Fein and Klarman maintain that unlike insurance companies or families, society as a whole is concerned with total output, of which consumption is the major component. They argue that man is not a machine, and consumption is the ultimate goal of economic activity. Accordingly, a net production after consumption is not relevant to the economists' central concern and consumption should not be deducted.

Weisbrod's position is that the treatment of consumption depends upon one's view of society—that is whether the potential survivor is regarded as a member. If he is, consumption should not be deducted from earnings, and conversely.[25] Although Weisbrod does not *explicitly* choose between the two views, he does develop elaborate and carefully calculated estimates of consumption expenditures (as a function of age) on the basis of household budget studies. These consumption estimates are deducted from output gains to obtain a net figure.

The medical care expenditures of a person in an institution automatically reduce his ordinary expenditures as a consumer. These should be deducted to the extent that his family reduces its own expenditures. The size of the reduction is likely to be greater for long-term than for short-term institutional care. In the short-term instance these expenditures are small and can be ignored.[26]

Housewives Services

Economists differ on the treatment of housewives' services in the calculation of the indirect costs of illness. Those who would exclude them from the calculations acknowledge that the result is a serious understatement of the costs of disease, but the exclusion is generally justified on two grounds: One is the difficulty of measuring the contribution of housewives to national income. Because this contribution occurs *outside the market*, the imputation (attributing the equivalent of a market price where none exists) of economic value raises many statistical problems.[27] The other is that to include the contribution of housewives is inconsistent with the accepted procedures of national income accounting.[28]

The second point is irrelevant; since the figures are not additive, the income loss associated with a particular disease is meant to be compared with a similar figure for another disease.

The first point is true. However, while the economic value of housewives' services is difficult to measure, trying to compute it does less harm than neglecting it. Specifically, to disregard the services of housewives in calculating output loss is to understate the benefits of any health program designed to serve a predominantly female population.

There are two major methods to determine the economic value of housewives.

1. *The opportunity cost of being a housewife.* Given her education, training, and age, how much would she earn in full-time employment? As in the case of wage workers one would also have to consider the value of fringe benefits in addition to actual wages received.

2. *The replacement cost of a housewife.* Weisbrod bases his measure of the value of a housewife on the size of the household to be cared for, the latter being a function of the age of the woman. Rice and others have more simply estimated the value of housewives' services at the level of earnings of a domestic servant. This amount is admittedly low since it makes no allowance for the housewives' longer work week and greater variety of tasks. Moreover, since most domestic servants are black, their earnings reflect discrimination based on race and sex.

Given the present distribution of education and earnings of the female population, the opportunity cost measure will yield a much higher figure for the economic value of housewives than the replacement cost measure.

Measurement of Intangibles

A common difficulty in measurement of the benefits of health services is that few (if any) health services are pure investment goods or consumption goods that yield the same degree of health improvement. It is common to recognize the consumption benefit derived from most health and medical care expenditures (such as reduction of pain, discomfort, and anxiety), to discuss the difficulty of measuring it, and then to ignore the issue.[29]

Klarman attempted to measure the consumption benefit associated with the eradication of syphilis. His approach was to consider an analogous disease, one which was deemed to produce nonpecuniary consequences that are of the same degree of severity as syphilis. Klarman writes:

Consider a disease B (with symptoms that are somewhat similar to those of disease A), for which medical care expenditures are incurred both without any prospect of a return in increased output (either because the disease is not disabling or because the patient has retired from the labor force) and without prospect of an offsetting reduction in medical care expenditures in the future (because the disease is not curable and expenditures do not cease). These expenditures are incurred for consumption purposes only, and by analogy they may be held to indicate the value of the consumption benefit attached to avoiding the disease A under study.[30]

Klarman argues that an analogous disease to infectious syphilis is psoriasis, a skin disease. The analogous disease for syphlitic psychoses is terminal cancer. Some physicians have strongly disagreed with Klarman's choice of analogous diseases, but as a minimum he has made a pioneering attempt to measure the consumer benefit associated with disease control.

**Cost-benefit Analysis in
Developing Countries**

The data requirements that are necessary to undertake a sophisticated cost-benefit study are severe. One requires information on earnings by age and sex, labor force participation and unemployment rates by age and sex; life tables, which permit calculation of the probability of living to retirement age, information on the direct expenditures for health services, as well as data on the distribution of deaths and morbidity by age and sex for the disease or diseases under consideration. Most of this information is simply not collected or available in developing countries, forcing researchers to make approximations or even guesses at the magnitudes of the parameters involved.

Moreover, agricultural and other subsistence level workers in many developing countries are often not a part of the cash economy, although they may occasionally engage in some market transactions. Nevertheless, they do engage in production and consumption of commodities and thus their premature mortality and morbidity has economic consequences. With much of the labor force in developing countries engaged in subsistence agriculture the measurement of the economic cost of disease for this group is a major and important challenge.

Finally, there is considerable evidence that chronic underemployment exists in many developing countries, especially in the agricultural regions. This may amount to as much as one-fourth of the labor force.[31] To determine the value of lost production due to premature mortality and morbidity given underemployment of this magnitude is an extremely difficult task.

D.H.S. Griffiths, et al., provide an interesting example of a cost-benefit study of malaria prophylaxis in a province of western Thailand. Tungsten is readily available in this region. The plentiful supply of ore and low capital costs of extraction had led a number of small entrepreneurs to retrieve the metal from the region's rivers. This is a highly profitable operation. However, in spite of the relatively high wages (800 baht per month), the labor force would only remain in the area a short time, primarily because of the extent and severity of malaria.

Data on the size of the labor force in 1969 is not available nor is information regarding the number of man-hours worked. However, the volume of production provides a clue. Until December 1969 production of tungsten in one particular enterprise was always less than 1,000 kg. per month. According to the owner, the average extraction rate by one man per month is about 75 kg. (or 3 kg. per day in a 25 day working month). This would put the equivalent full-time labor force at 10 man-equivalents per month if it is assumed that the total output averaged 750 kg. per month for each month until December 1969.[32] When malaria prophylaxis was introduced, the turnover of labor decreased and the total labor force increased. In December 1969 production reached 1,000 kg. In January 1970 it became 2,000 kg. and in February and March it was maintained each month at approximately 3,000 kg.

One can estimate the profits accruing to this medical effort, particularly the possible increase due to the malaria prophylaxis. The cost of extraction, transportation, and sale in bahts (Bt.) per kilogram are indicated in Table 5-2.

Assuming that output would have remained at 750 kg. per month, the return for August 1969 to March 1970 would have been (750 kg. × 8 × Bt. 45) = Bt. 270,000.

If the difference in estimated output with and without malaria prophylaxis is

Table 5-2

Costs and Returns on Tungsten Production, Kanchanaburi Province, Thailand

Item	Cost
Labor cost per Kg.	Bt. 11
Government taxes per Kg.	Bt. 10
Transportation to Kanchanaburi	Bt. 1
Other expenditures	Bt. 8
Total cost to Kanchanaburi	Bt. 30 per Kg.
Estimated value of Tungsten at Kanchanaburi	Bt. 75 per Kg.
Estimated return on production of 1 Kg.	Bt. 45 per Kg.
Estimated total cost, August 1969 to March 1970	Bt. 360,000
Estimated value August 1960 to March 1970	Bt. 900,000
Estimated total return on production	Bt. 540,000

Source: D.H.S. Griffith, D.V. Ramana, and H. Mashaal, "Contribution of Health to Development," *International Journal of Health Services*, Vol. 1, No. 3, August 1971, p. 269. Copyright Baywood Publishing Co., Inc., 1971.

then regarded as the "benefit" that was gained, it is easy to see that the value of this can be estimated at 270,000 baht. This is because the total return on production for the eight-month period was in fact $540,000 and would have been only $270,000 if the malaria prophylaxis had not been introduced.

Moreover, the total expenditure on malaria prophylaxis can be estimated at a maximum of 225 baht per worker per month. Assuming a total expenditure of 225 X 4 months X 40 workers or 36,000 baht and a value of benefit for the period December to March of 270,000 baht, a direct cost-benefit ratio for this period can be determined. First, it is necessary to deduct the expenditure on drugs from the benefit. This leaves 234,000 baht. Dividing this now by the drug expenditure, it would appear that the direct cost-benefit ratio for the period December to March was equivalent to 1:6.50. It should be noted that the increase in benefit was not caused by an increase in per capita output, but was due to a total increase and stabilization of the labor force.

Stephen Enke has pioneered in the application of cost-benefit analysis to the problem of population size. He has developed estimates of the cost and present benefits to society of preventing births.[33]

A basic element in such an analysis is a calculation of the economic value of preventing one birth. By subtracting the lifetime consumption from lifetime product for a marginal birth in India, he determined the former would exceed the latter by 6,000 rupees.[34]

Enke then refined his calculations by introducing a rate of discount. He selected 10 percent as the discount rate and pointed out that since the newly born individual will not begin producing for 15 years, the discounted present value of his production is almost zero. However, because the person will begin consuming immediately the present discounted value of his consumption will not be negligible. For India he estimated it to be 690 rupees. Thus, in India the costs of consumption associated with one additional individual exceed the value of his production implying that a lower birth rate would result in a net economic gain.

This methodological approach can be criticized from several points of view. First, the actual costs of a child fall on its parents and perhaps also on older children. Additional children per family lower the available average subsistence per family member but it is less clear that the additional births affect society as a whole. Indeed, it can be argued that children are a special type of asset for parents, generating a future stream of real economic benefits (support in old age of the parents, unpaid labor in the family farm, dowry income at the time of marriage), and that they also provide direct "consumption" satisfaction, from the enjoyment of having offspring. Thus, if parents accept the apparent "costs" in the form of reduced consumption, of an additional child, the choice may represent a welfare maximizing course of action from their viewpoint.[35]

Criticisms of Cost-benefit Analyses of Health Programs

A number of criticisms have been directed at the cost-benefit approach to program planning. First, it provides inadequate rationale or guidance in health programs for the poor. Our reasons, as a society, for undertaking programs to aid the poor are becoming increasingly complex, but it is clear that profitability is at most a minor consideration.[36] Use of human capital concepts will generally yield the conclusion that less should be spent on the poor (since they earn less money) than is spent on the rich. But the conclusion that poverty health programs should be small is clearly contrary to current public desire and public policy. However, cost-benefit analysis could be of help in choosing among alternative poverty programs or in attempting to decide what are the desirable components of any specific program.

Moreover, the lack of relevance of such calculations is illustrated by the fact that Medicare was the program that opened the door to major participation by the United States government in payment for medical care. Human-capital calculations would indicate that medical care to persons over 65 is relatively unimportant, but politicians know that such care was very important not only to the recipients but to the (voting-age) children of the recipients. Moreover, the major program proposed by the administration in 1968 (a time when cost-benefit analysis and cost-effectiveness analysis was used widely in program planning) was the maternal and child health programs, even though women and children have relatively low expected earnings.

However, such criticism of cost-benefit analysis as that rendered above is to some extent naive. One must always remember that political realities may well dominate cost-benefit calculations in determining priorities. For example, fluoridation was shown to have a very high benefit-to-cost ratio, but it was replaced in the Johnson administration's legislative proposal by a more expensive and less effective treatment program because of fear of those opposed to flouridation.[37] One must always remember that cost-benefit calculations are but one element (albeit an important one) in the decision-making process.

Brian Abel-Smith argues that to be really useful, cost-benefit analysis of health programs requires a measure of health output.

We need to be able to specify in precise quantitative form what we are trying to achieve so that we can establish a relationship between input and output—between blocks of expenditure and measured steps towards the attainment of these objectives. There are, however, few fields where output is so hard to measure as it is in health services. We can within limits measure inputs—the resources of manpower and goods which are used in health services. . . . We can measure the quantity of services which are provided in units, such as patients treated, persons immunized, or area sprayed, but these activities which we record are only means to an end which is the improvement of health."[38]

Moreover, health programs are only one method of improving health. The health of a population depends on many other factors, such as nutrition and environment, which are not normally considered part of the health sector. Nevertheless, if we are to measure the output of health services, we will need to determine the contribution the latter factors make to health status. This is clearly a formidable task.

Finally, because of complexities and uncertainties, there must be a large element of qualitative analysis, as well as the quantitative methods stressed above. One of the dangers of using the cost-benefit method is that analysts and decision makers become so enthralled with the apparent precise answers it produces that they may forget the oversimplifying assumptions that were necessary to arrive at the quantitative solution.[39]

Cost-effectiveness Analysis

Cost-effectiveness analysis differs from cost-benefit analysis in that costs are calculated and alternative ways are compared for achieving *a specific set of results.* Our objective is not just how to use funds most efficiently, it also includes the constraint that a specified output must be achieved. Very often, this output is not expressed in dollars.[40] Cost-benefit studies expedite comparisons among several programs with differing objectives, whereas cost-effectiveness analysis is used in a comparison of different ways of reaching the same objective. In both cost-benefit and cost-effectiveness studies, one is limited because there is no satisfactory unit of measurement common to the benefits from various health programs.

From a managerial standpoint cost-effectiveness analysis is directed by two basic economic considerations: (1) that for the program being considered there will be a dollar of return for each dollar of investment, returns being measured in either social or economic terms; (2) that optimally the program's return (in either social or economic terms) will be greater than expenditures.[41]

Example of a Cost-effectiveness Study

A study of cost-effectiveness in maternal and child health had as its general objective making needed maternal and child health services available and accessible to all, and particularly to all expectant mothers and children in "health depressed areas."[42] In addition, three subordinate objectives were proposed: (1) to reduce infant mortality rates; (2) to reduce unmet dental needs; and (3) to reduce the incidence of preventable handicapping conditions and the prevalence of uncorrected handicapping conditions in children.

Cost estimates for all programs included costs for renovation of equipment prorated over a 10 year period, and yearly diagnostic treatment costs. Manpower costs were predicated upon utilization of three new types of health workers— obstetric and pediatric assistants and dental auxiliaries.

Arranging the several programs that were considered beside their respective effects per $10,000,000 of program cost allows a rapid comparison of what may be expected from each program—its relative cost effectiveness. (See Table 5-3.) From Table 5-3 it can be seen, for instance, that a program to expand family-planning services to reach an additional one-half million women in health depressed areas would be about five and one half times as cost-effective in reducing yearly infant deaths as a program to provide intensive care units for high-risk newborn infants. Comprehensive care would be considerably less cost-effective in this regard than either of the other alternatives. Similarly Table 5-3 indicates that periodic case finding and treatment programs would be several times as cost-effective in preventing or correcting certain handicapping conditions as comprehensive care would be, although the case finding programs would not display many of the other benefits of comprehensive care such as a reduction in maternal and infant deaths. In reducing the amount of unmet dental needs, a flouridation program appears to be the most cost-effective, and is much more so than if it were combined with a program of comprehensive dental care.

T. Paul Schultz has used cost-effectiveness analysis to evaluate various aspects of the family planning program in Taiwan. One aspect of the program that he analyzed was the mix of personnel. Discussion here deals only with the trade-off between village health education nurses (VHEN) and prepregnancy health workers (PPHW), whose training and salaries are roughly comparable. Regression analysis indicates that the use of the village health education nurse has about double the impact on birth rates as does the prepregnancy health worker.[43] This

Table 5-3
Summary of Estimated Yearly Effects of Alternative Child Health Care Programs, Per $10,000,000 Expended in Health-depressed Areas

Program	No. Served	Births Prevented	Maternal Deaths Prevented	Premature Births Prevented	Infant Deaths Prevented
Comprehensive health care (up to age 18)	3,500 mothers 63,000 children	0	1.6	98-247	42-60
Comprehensive health care (up to age 5)	6,880 mothers 34,400 children	0	3	196-483	84-119
Case finding & treatment (newborn infants)	337,000 screened 12,470 treated	—	—	—	—
Case finding & treatment (ages 0,1,3,5, & 9)	334,000 screened (39,000 treated)	—	—	—	—
Vision & hearing case finding & treatment	1,458,000 screened (63,000 treated)	—	—	—	—
Fluoridation	14,112,000 aged 0-12	—	—	—	—
Comprehensive dental care (without fluoridation)	33,000 aged 6-18	—	—	—	—
Comprehensive dental care & fluoridation	1,200,000 aged 0-18	—	—	—	—
Intensive-care units for high-risk newborn infants	10,710	—	—	—	367
Expanded family-planning services	500,000	49,000	44	—	2,000

Program	Mental Retardation Prevented	Vision Problems		Hearing Loss		Other Physical Handicaps	Unmet Dental Needs
		All	Amblyopia	All	Binaural		
Comprehensive health care (up to age 18)	4.5-7	345	59	86	7.2	200	2,240
Comprehensive health care (up to age 5)	7-14	196	.119	70	4.9	63	0
Case finding & treatment (newborn infants)	—	—	—	—	—	—	—
Case finding & treatment (ages 0,1,3,5 & 9)	—	3,610	1,140	1,000	60	1,470	—
Vision & hearing case finding & treatment	—	26,250	8,260	4,370	437	—	—
Fluoridation	—	—	—	—	—	—	294,000
Comprehensive dental care (without fluoridation)	—	—	—	—	—	—	18,000
Comprehensive dental care & fluoridation	—	—	—	—	—	—	44,000
Intensive-care units for high-risk newborn infants	—	—	—	—	—	—	—
Expanded family-planning services	1,000	—	—	—	—	—	—

Source: U.S. Department of Health, Education, and Welfare, Office of the Assistant Secretary for Program Coordination, *Program Analysis: Maternal and Child Health Programs* (Washington, D.C.: U.S. Government Printing Office, 1966), p. iv 10.

implies that since it costs about the same to hire either class of field worker, with more VHEN and fewer PPHW the program would appear to have elicited a greater reduction in birth rates than actually occurred, lowering the average and marginal program cost per birth overted.

Concerns have been expressed about the exclusion of nonquantifiable factors when undertaking cost-effectiveness analyses. A.R. Prest and Ralph Turvey have warned against the analyst's tendency to structure alternatives in terms of data availability. They caution that many of the differences in estimating benefits "stem from differences in the availability of statistics, rather than from differences in what the authors would like to measure if they could."[44]

Cost-effectiveness analysis should serve to make the analyst aware of a lack of basic information on program effectiveness. Thus, it should encourage health professionals not only to develop measures of effectiveness but also to structure alternatives which consider widely varying combinations of resources.

Summary

Cost-benefit analysis of health programs has as its historical antecedent attempts to measure the capitalized value of human life. The total economic costs of illness are comprised of two elements, the direct expenditures for medical treatment and the indirect costs of illness that include morbidity, premature mortality, and pain and suffering. In a cost-benefit analysis the comparison is between expected additional expenditures for health services and the anticipated reduction in present costs.

A number of methodological issues that arise in a cost-benefit analysis of health programs were discussed, such as the choice of discount rate, the calculation of output loss, and the valuation of housewives' services. Several of these issues are presently unresolved.

Cost-effectiveness analysis examines the most efficient way of achieving a given objective. Frequently the objective is not expressed in dollar terms but in terms of a given health measure, such as "years of life saved." Cost-effectiveness studies are frequently constrained by lack of data on effectiveness measures.

Cost-benefit and cost-effectiveness analysis provide important insights regarding the choice of alternatives. However, political as well as social factors will always play an important role in decision making.

Notes

1. Royal A. Crystal and Agnes W. Brewster, "Cost-Benefit and Cost-Effectiveness Analyses in the Health Field: An Introduction," *Inquiry*, Vol. III, No. 4, December 1966, p. 4.

2. Warren Smith, "Cost-Effectiveness and Cost-Benefit Analyses for Public Health Programs," *Public Health Reports*, Vol. 83, No. 11, November 1968, p. 899.

3. Henry Bixby Hemenway, "Economics of Health Administration," *American Journal of Public Health*, Vol. 10, No. 2, February, 1920, pp. 105-6.

4. Sir William Petty, *Political Arithmetick, or a Discourse Concerning the Extent and Value of Lands, People, Buildings, Etc.* (London: Robert Clavel, 1699).

5. Ibid.

6. Edwin Chadwick, *Report on the Sanitary Conditions of the Laboring Population of Great Britain* (London: W. Clowes and Sons for H.M. Stationery Office, 1842).

7. Chadwick, *Report*, p. 275.

8. William Farr, "The Income and Property Tax," *Journal of the Statistical Society*, Vol. 16, March 1853, pp. 41-44.

9. Max Von Pettenkofer, *The Value of Health to a City.* Translated from the German, with an Introduction by Henry E. Sigerist (Baltimore, Maryland: The Johns Hopkins Press, 1941).

10. Mark Perlman, "On Health and Economic Development: Some Problems, Methods and Conclusions Reviewed in a Perusal of the Literature," *Comparative Studies in Society and History*, Vol. 8, 1966, p. 435.

11. Irving Fisher, *Report on National Vitality, Its Wastes and Conservation* (Washington, D.C.: U.S. Government Printing Office, 1909), p. 120.

12. Burton Weisbrod, *Economics of Public Health* (Philadelphia, Pennsylvania: University of Pennsylvania Press, 1961), p. 90.

13. Dorothy Rice, "Estimating the Cost of Illness," *American Journal of Public Health*, Vol. 57, No. 3, March 1967, p. 437.

14. Weisbrod, *Economics*, p. 33.

15. Herbert E. Klarman, "Socio-Economic Impact of Heart Disease," in *The Heart and Circulation: Second National Conference on Cardiovascular Diseases* (Washington, D.C.: U.S. Government Printing Office, 1964), Vol. II, Chapter 2, p. 699.

16. Maynard M. Hufschmidt, *Standards and Criteria for Formulating and Evaluating Federal Water Resources Developments* (Washington, D.C.: U.S. Bureau of the Budget, 1961), p. 11; and Stephen A. Marglin, "Economic Factors Affecting System Design," in Arthur Maass, et al., *Design of Water Resource Systems* (Cambridge, Massachusetts: Harvard University Press, 1962), p. 194.

17. Martin S. Feldstein, "Review of Weisbrod's Economics of Public Health," *Economic Journal*, Vol. 73, March 1963, pp. 129-30.

18. Herbert E. Klarman, "Syphilis Control Programs," in Robert Dorfman (Ed.), *Measuring Benefits of Public Investments* (Washington, D.C.: The Brookings Institution, 1965), p. 373.

19. See for example, Rashi Fein, *The Economics of Mental Illness* (New

York: Basic Books, 1958), p. 73; and John Krutilla and Otto Eckstein, *Multiple Purpose River Development* (Baltimore, Maryland: The Johns Hopkins Press, 1958), Chapter 4.

20. U.S. Congress, Joint Economic Committee, Subcommittee on Economy in Government, 90th Congress, 1st Session, *The Planning-Programming-Budgeting System: Progress and Potentials* (Washington, D.C.: U.S. Government Printing Office, 1967), p. 160.

21. Robert L. Banks and Arnold Katz, "The Program Budget and the Interest Rate for Public Investment," *Public Administration Review*, Vol. 26, No. 6, December 1966, pp. 283-92.

22. Klarman, "Syphilis Control Programs," p. 374.

23. Eli Ginzberg, "Health, Medicine, and Economic Welfare," *Journal of the Mount Sinai Hospital*, Vol. 19, March-April 1953, pp. 734-43.

24. Louis I. Dublin and Alfred J. Lotka, *The Money Value of a Man*, rev. ed. (New York: Ronald Press, 1946), p. 77.

25. See Weisbrod, *Economics*, pp. 35-36, for a more detailed discussion of this point.

26. Klarman, "Syphilis Control Programs," p. 381.

27. Fein, *The Economics of Mental Illness*, pp. 23-24 and p. 143.

28. Selma J. Mushkin and Francis d'A. Collings, "Economic Costs of Disease and Injury," *Public Health Reports*, Vol. 74, No. 9, September 1959, pp. 803-4.

29. Fein, *The Economics of Mental Illness*, p. 29; Rice, "Estimating the Cost of Illness," p. 429; and D.J. Reynolds, "The Cost of Road Accidents," *Journal of the Royal Statistical Society*, Vol. 119, 1956, Part IV, pp. 393-408.

30. Klarman, "Syphilis Control Programs," p. 371.

31. N.S. Buchanan and H.S. Ellis, *Approaches to Economic Development* (New York: Twentieth Century Fund, 1955), p. 45.

32. D.H.S. Griffith, D.V. Ramana, and H. Marshaal, "Contribution of Health to Development," *International Journal of Health Services*, Vol. I, No. 3, August 1971, p. 269.

33. Stephen Enke, "The Economic Aspects of Slowing Population Growth," *The Economic Journal*, Vol. 76, March 1966, pp. 44-56.

34. Stephen Enke, "The Gains to India from Population Control: Some Money Measures and Incentive Schemes," *Review of Economics and Statistics*, Vol. 42, No. 3, May 1960, p. 176.

35. Warren C. Robinson and David E. Horlacher, *Population Growth and Economic Welfare*, Reports on Population/Family Planning (New York: The Population Council, February 1971), p. 6.

36. Vincent D. Taylor, "How Much is Good Health Worth?" (Santa Monica, California: Rand Corp., unpublished, MS, P-3945, October 1968), p. 7.

37. Elizabeth B. Drew, "HEW Grapples with PPBS," *Public Interest*, Vol. 7, Summer, 1967, p. 27.

38. Brian Abel-Smith, "Health Priorities in Developing Countries: The Econo-

mists Contribution," *International Journal of Health Services*, Vol. 2, No. 1, February 1972, pp. 6-7. Copyright Baywood Publishing Co., Inc., 1972.

39. David F. Bergwall, Philip N. Reeves, and Nina B. Woodside, *Introduction to Health Planning* (Washington, D.C.: Information Resources Press, 1974), p. 179.

40. Warren Smith, "Cost-Effectiveness and Cost-Benefit Analyses," pp. 899-900.

41. Crystal and Brewster, "Cost-Benefit and Cost-Effectiveness Analyses," p. 8.

42. Arthur L. Levin, "Cost Effectiveness in Maternal and Child Health: Implications for Program Planning and Evaluation," *New England Journal of Medicine*, Vol. 278, No. 19, May 9, 1968, p. 1042.

43. T. Paul Schultz, "The Effectiveness of Family Planning in Taiwan: A Proposal for a New Evaluation Methodology," unpublished manuscript, 1969, the Rand Corp., p. 52.

44. A.R. Prest and Ralph Turvey, Cost Benefit Analysis: Survey in American Economic Association. *Surveys of Economic Theory: Prepared for the Association and the Royal Economic Society*, Vol. 2, Survey 8 (New York: St. Martins Press, 1966), p. 158.

6

Health, Population, and Economic Development in Developing Countries

The associations between health and national development are complex. The interaction is a two-way phenomenon, with health being both influenced by and influencing economic development. Improved health for too long has been considered solely a result of economic growth, a part of the product of growth rather than one of its causes.

Some development experts have maintained that health should have low priority in development funding and have justified their opinions with comments such as, "Only a rich nation can afford the programs to assure its population's health," or "A poor nation cannot afford improved health." The concern of development planners is accentuated by the fact that during the demographic transition lower death rates are often associated with sustained high birth rates, which results in rapid population growth. For example, in Ceylon the death rate fell from 20.2 per 1,000 in 1946 to 10.1 in 1954.[1] Since the birth rate remained constant at 35 to 40 per 1,000 the rate of population growth nearly doubled. The widespread utilization of low-cost public health measures, including malaria eradication, played a significant role in the swift decline in mortality rates.[2]

While the supply of labor may increase in quantity and quality from improved health and reduced death rates, there may be no corresponding gain in per capita output. Thus, if economic growth is too slow to absorb the additions to the labor force associated with expanded health programs, greater unemployment, both open and disguised, may result. Thus, improved health in poor societies can be postulated to produce larger populations, greater poverty, and ultimately deterioration in health.

However, other development planners and economists are more optimistic regarding the impact of health and nutrition programs on economic growth. There are three different ways by which improved health programs can accelerate development. First, improved health may increase the productivity or efficiency of the labor force, leading to greater output and reduced cost per unit. Second, better health conditions may serve to open new regions of a country for settlement and subsequent development. Finally, attitudinal changes toward achievement and entrepreneurship may be linked to health and nutrition programs. This linkage, which is virtually unexplored, has major significance because of the importance of stimulating entrepreneurship in poor countries. Empirical studies concerning the importance of these three kinds of relationships between health and development are considered.

It has become apparent that where health conditions are worst, relatively simple and low-cost health programs can produce dramatic lessening of debility and disability of the labor force. In these situations major increments in productivity are most readily apparent.[3] For example, in the Philippines in 1946 a survey of major enterprises indicated a daily absenteeism rate of 35 percent, attributed largely to malaria. After initiation of an antimalaria program, the rate of absenteeism was reduced to between 2 and 4 percent, and nearly one-fourth fewer laborers were required for any given task.[4] In southern Rhodesia, an antimalaria campaign reduced absenteeism during the harvest season in the Mazoe Valley from 25 percent to almost negligible levels.[5] In Haiti, where yaws was widely prevalent among the rural population, 35,000 to 50,000 persons were treated monthly in a joint World Health Organization-UNICEF campaign. It was estimated that 100,000 incapacitated persons returned to work.[6] B.A. Weisbrod and his colleagues, in a recent extensive study in St. Lucia regarding the effects of schistosomiasis (as well as other parasitic diseases) on productivity, failed to find any association between the severity of the disease and the fertility of women, the educational achievement of children, and the daily output of workers on a banana plantation.[7] Some observers have questioned whether schistosomiasis is severe enough on St. Lucia to result in lower productivity. Moreover, the study measured the effect of the disease on the learning of those in school and at work. The researchers thus ignored those persons too sick to work or too ill to attend school.

A number of studies have linked individual output to health or nutritional status. H.A. Kraut and E.A. Muller indicated the association between calorie consumption and personal productivity. In one case 20 workmen were building an embankment by dumping debris from railroad cars. While receiving a diet supplying only 820 calories per day over the 1,600 to 1,800 calories needed for resting metabolism, they dumped 1.5 tons of debris per hour. When they were provided a diet designed for workers in heavy industry, their output increased to 2.2 tons per hour.[8] An equally dramatic increase in output per worker occurred when laborers constructing the Pan American Highway began receiving three well-balanced meals daily.[9]

Is there any way of determining quantitatively the increased productivity required to outweigh the negative economic effect of population increase? Little hard research has been undertaken in this area but preliminary estimates have been made on the basis of econometric models.[10] For example, Selma Mushkin has estimated the increase in real gross national product resulting from disease eradication. She assumed that a disease such as malaria affected 80 percent of the population of an agricultural area, prevalence being uniform among men, women, and children. She also assumed that the morbidity associated with malaria reduced the productivity of agricultural workers by 30 percent during a three-month period when the disease was at its peak. The output loss was calculated to be 6 percent within the agricultural sector. If agriculture accounted for one-third of the total output, elimination of the productivity loss attributable to malaria would increase the gross national product by 1.0 percent.[11]

If the disease exerted its debilitating effect for the whole year rather than for three months, as would be the case, for example, with schistosomiasis, the increase in national output that would result from its elimination could be as great as 4.0 percent.[12] Paul Enterline and William Stewart estimated that an increase in life expectancy at birth from 30 to 32.5 years would require an increase of 0.8 percent in output per worker to maintain per capita income. (They assumed a marginal capital-output ratio of 3 to 1.)[13] Using this estimate Mushkin concluded that if eradication of a disease increased life expectancy at birth by 2.5 years, gains in total output due to reductions in morbidity would exceed by a considerable margin the 0.8 percent increase required to maintain the existing level of per capita income.

As indicated earlier, there is some likelihood that increases in productivity and declines in absenteeism that result from public health programs may result in additional unemployment. This will occur if workers displaced by productivity gains in one sector of the economy do not find jobs in another sector, or if demand for the product is inelastic so that price decreases associated with productivity gains do not stimulate any major changes in the quantity demanded and concomitantly the number of workers required to produce the product. For example, there is the case of Mexican village potters who suffered lead intoxication from the oxide used in glazing. A United Nations program to combat the "saturnismo" did improve health and did expand worker effectiveness and output. In the absence of other inputs, unemployment was aggravated when the industry's economic position was depressed by excess supplies.[14]

Health and Regional Development

Health programs can affect the rate of growth of regional development. For example, the introduction of a major health program can stimulate the settlement and development of areas where economic activity had previously been impossible because of adverse health conditions. The upsurge in economic activity will tend to encourage migration from overcrowded and depressed areas and can result in an increase in *total* employment as well as a sharp rise in gross regional product.

There has been little *systematic* research on the impact of health on regional development. Much of the literature is provided by noneconomists so that a suitable analytic framework is lacking in most of the studies. Thus, much of the literature is purely descriptive. With the exception of a few summary statistics, there has been little focus on the kind of development that has occurred.

During the 1940s and 1950s widespread malaria eradication campaigns in parts of Asia and Africa resulted in many cases of accelerated regional development. For example, the severe hyperendemic malaria of the Terai forests below the Himalayan foothills had made the Rapti Valley of Nepal virtually uninhabitable for centuries. After a widespread mosquito control program was undertaken during the 1950s, this fertile valley was opened up for settlers from densely populated Nepalese hillsides. By the late 1960s, the population of the valley had increased tenfold and economic activity in the agricultural and extractive industries was increasing rapidly.[15]

A malaria eradication program has enabled an area in central Thailand that was previously sparsely inhabited and yielded little in agricultural production to undergo profound economic change. By 1957, 7,000 families had settled in the region and the value of total agricultural production had reached $35 million.[16]

In Ghana onchocerciasis (river blindness) had driven farmers from the fertile north to the less fertile central and southern regions of the country.

All along the retreating frontier of settlement there is a pervading atmosphere of decline and decay. Few of the houses are well maintained; although land is abundant, farms are not large and tend to be neglected because of limitations on the labor force, many of whom are blind. To the lay observer, nutritional standards seem to be low, and the incidence of minor infections such as sores, is much higher than in the interior. When one visits these small, isolated and dying communities, one cannot help feeling the contrast between the vigor and energy of the central and western sections, and the lethargy and quiet resignation on the border of the blind area.[17]

Beginning along the Red Volta, where the incidence of onchocerciasis was greatest, land has been abandoned at the rate of one mile every 7 to 14 years for the past 45 to 50 years.[18] While other diseases may have played a role, the primary agent is indisputably river blindness.

The economic development of very extensive areas, particularly in the savannahs of tropical Africa, cannot occur without first controlling onchocerciasis. This situation is most serious in certain West African states such as Mali and Upper Volta, where the greater part of the fertile land is in areas where the disease is firmly established. Following requests for assistance by the governments concerned, the Volta River Basin, an area of 700,000 square kilometers comprising parts of seven countries, Upper Volta, Niger, Ivory Coast, Mali, Togo, Dahomey, and Ghana, has been chosen as the first area for control under a WHO sponsored project.

Investment Priorities

In most of the instances in which disease control has accelerated regional development, the major purpose of the health program was humanitarian. For example, regarding malaria, systematic consideration of the economic potential of the areas where spraying was carried out was not undertaken; as a result, control was frequently carried out in regions of both low and high economic expectations. An important exception to the policy has been Kenya, where the government has tended to concentrate antimalarial and other public health measures in areas having high growth possibilities.[19] Moreover, malaria eradication in Ethiopia has been concentrated in areas where the outlook for economic development was favorable. Thus, eradication has been concentrated in the Awash River Valley as well as the rich Kobbo-Chercher plain.[20]

Ruderman has criticized the policy of concentrating health expenditures in the most potentially productive regions.[21] First, it may not be politically feasible to limit public health programs to certain geographical areas. Second, the nature of communicable diseases implies that although treatment can take place on an individual basis, control can be realized only on an unselective community basis. Finally, he argues that selective health programs can take place only after basic health services are already well developed as a result of earlier investment decisions. This basic health infrastructure does not exist in much of Asia, Africa, and Latin America.

Health Programs and Attitude Changes

There is the possibility that a health measure may be associated with economic gains primarily because of changes in the motivation and attitudes of the workers toward the feasibility of improvement in the overall quality of life. For example, Wilfred Malenbaum suggests that health inputs in physical facilities have a high demonstration effect on the power of man to influence his own destiny. For the bulk of the poor, and especially the poor peasant, the difficulties of life often tend to be accepted as predestined. Health programs may serve to challenge the notion of the inevitability of poverty and powerlessness. Since the consequences of new health facilities are highly visible, the peasant's own decisions on other matters, and especially on economic activities, may begin to reflect a new way of thinking about the future. In a sense he begins to feel that he is able to influence events. His knowledge of the power of health services and of his capacity to avail himself of them constitutes direct evidence that his decisions do influence his own prospects in this life. Indeed, some consequences of this new potential may be expected initially in directions other than those where customs, superstition, and religion hold greatest sway.[22] Thus, the effects of attitudinal change may be first manifested in an expanded output of goods and increased entrepreneurial activity rather than, for example, in smaller sized families.

There is one important dimension of the mental aspects of poor health that must be considered; this is the consequence of inadequate protein intake for the unborn fetus as well as for infants and young children. The damage done by deterred brain development due to protein malnutrition and maternal neglect may be irreparable after the child is two or three years old.[23] Appropriate nutrition and feeding programs can thus result in a labor force with a larger proportion of mentally alert adults. Such a labor force is more likely to include individuals capable of growth contributing activities than one with a higher degree of malnutrition.

Malenbaum tested the above propositions on the basis of macroeconomic (countrywide) data for 22 poor countries as well as regional data for India, Thailand, and Mexico. In all cases agricultural output was employed as the dependent variable, with various health, economic, and social measures serving as independent variables.

Using a step wise regression equation, Malenbaum obtained the following results from the countrywide data:[24]

$$X_1 = 133 + 0.344X_2 + 0.038X_3 - 0.13X_4 - 0.00095X_5 - 0.024X_6$$
$$[2.2] \qquad [0.73] \qquad [2.7] \qquad [3.8] \qquad [0.25]$$

where X_1 refers to agricultural output; X_2 agricultural labor; X_3 commercial fertilizer; X_4 infant mortality; X_5 the physician population ratio; and X_6 illiteracy. (The figures in brackets are the elasticities calculated at the means of the variables.)

The five independent variables account for over 62 percent of all the variation in output among countries. Of the total variation explained, about one-fifth comes from the agricultural variables and almost four-fifths from the health variables; less than 2 percent comes from the degree of literacy.[25]

The data for the developing areas as national units do provide evidence of statistically significant relationships between production and health; moreover, the influence of health factors on output appears to be much larger in comparison with the importance of other variables including agricultural inputs. The degree of intercorrelation among the independent variables is small.

Table 6-1 compares Malenbaum's findings for Mexico, Thailand, and India with those discussed above.

Although the results are approximate, a health-output relationship does appear in all the areas investigated. While the question of the direction of this relationship cannot be resolved by statistics alone (health→ output vs. output→ health), the data in each case do suggest that the latter relationship is weaker than the former. For example, the programs for improved health through malaria control, infant mortality reduction, and better health facilities seem to have been initiated by the central authorities purely on the basis of social concern and not as a result of economic progress.

These relationships were observed in areas where the supply of labor is relatively abundant and where the supply of other factors of production have not been increased as a result of health programs. This implies that health-input production-output relation is affected in some measure by changes in motives and attitudes. In other words, as indicated above, health programs act to stimulate entrepreneurial activity.

The policy implications of these findings are fairly clear. If one expands

Table 6-1
Determinants of Output in Agriculture

Case	Output	R^2	Percentage of Covariation Associated with Inputs		
			Economic	Health	Other
Developing nations: 22 countries	Changes in agricultural output	0.62	20	79	1
Mexico: 1940 1960	Output per worker in agriculture	.66 .63	1 20	28 40	71 40
Thailand: 50 Provinces	Output per worker in agriculture	.62	85	5	10
India: 20 Blocks	Agricultural output	0.73	85	14	1

Source: Wilfred Malenbaum, "Health and Productivity in Poor Areas," in Herbert E. Klarman (Ed.), *Empirical Studies in Health Economics* (Baltimore, Maryland: The Johns Hopkins Press, © 1970), p. 49.

public health activities and therefore increases the supply of health manpower, there will be positive effects on output. In addition, there will likely be reductions in death rates and an increase in the rate of population growth for some time. However, if the effort to greater output is linked to attitude change as well as exploitation of resources, the growth of population will not automatically offset the expansion of output. Indeed, attitudes favoring individual progress should gradually serve to slow down the rate of population growth. Finally, to be most effective, the medical services also need to be combined with other goods and services—whether these be education or sanitation, or economic and social improvement programs.

Weisbrod and his associates have two major criticisms of Malenbaum's work. First, they indicate that because some of his health measures are inputs while others are outputs, the regression equations are not correctly specified. Thus, one cannot determine very clearly which health variables actually have a major impact on productivity.[26] Second, the measure of labor input employed is the percentage of the labor force in agriculture, which they contend is too imprecise a measure.[27]

Population Growth and Economic Development

The growth of the world's population has been at a dramatically increasing rate. Nearly 18 centuries passed before the population of the earth increased from a quarter to one billion persons. The next doubling took 130 years, with the world's population reaching approximately 2 billion by 1930. Since then the rise has been far more rapid with the number reaching 3.8 billion in 1974, and, if present growth rates are not changed, this figure will increase to approximately 7 billion by the year 2000.[28]

Death rates in developing countries have fallen greatly and can be expected to decline further. Moreover, because opportunities for emigration are much more limited than was the case in the nineteenth and earlier part of the twentieth century, economists and demographers have considered the effect of lower birth rates as a means of reducing the rate of population growth and increasing development.

A model developed by A.J. Coale and E.M. Hoover was used to estimate the effect of reduced fertility on income per consumer in India.

The heart of the model is a linear difference equation:

$$Y_t + 2.5 = Y_t + \frac{2.5G}{R}$$

where Y refers to real national income, G refers to adjusted gross investment, and R is the capital-output ratio. Let I equal annual investment and K total capital stock.

If we interpret G as equivalent to I or ΔK and R as $\frac{\Delta K}{\Delta Y}$ then:

$$\frac{G}{R} = (\Delta K) \div \frac{\Delta K}{\Delta Y} = \Delta Y$$

and, thus, the equation reduces to a statement that income in $t + 2.5$ years is equal to income in $t + 2.5$ times the annual growth rate, which depends on the level of investment and the capital-output ratio.[29]

In order to determine the equilibrium level of income and investment, Coale and Hoover implicitly equate savings and investment and introduce the following savings function:[30]

$$I = S = P\left[\frac{Io}{Po} + a\left(\frac{Y}{P} - \frac{Yo}{Po}\right)\right]$$

Thus, total savings are equal to population multiplied by per capita savings. Per capita savings are assumed to be equal to per capita investment in the base period plus a change in per capita savings induced by a change in per capita income. Coale and Hoover assume that the change in per capita savings is a constant proportion, a, of the change in per capita income from the base period.

By algebraic manipulation the terms of this equation may be rearranged so that it becomes:

$$I = aY - (\frac{aYo}{Po} - Io)P = Y - BP$$

In this form it is clear that investment is a linear function of income, assuming that population size, P, is demographically determined.[31]

Coale and Hoover applied the model to India and examined the change in income per consumer assuming a 50 percent reduction in the birth rate over a 30 year period.[32] They found that after 30 years income per adult consumer would be 38 to 45 percent higher if fertility were reduced by 50 percent than had fertility remained unchanged.

This result is not surprising. There are a variety of reasons why income per consumer can be expected to increase more rapidly when the birth rate is declining. First, a smaller population implies that the national income is shared by fewer persons. The national income itself is not reduced and in fact may be increased in the short run since the reduction in fertility does not lower the productive capacity of the economy.

Second, one can expect an increase in the rate of investment because a reduction in fertility increases the ability of a country to save. This result occurs because smaller families are able to divert a greater proportion of income from consumption expenditures to savings than larger families. This diversion of funds can occur either voluntarily through private savings, or involuntarily through government taxation. These increases in savings represent a potential source for the more rapid growth of investment and national income but the question arises whether parents, in fact, will increase savings or, alternatively, will consume all their increased (per capita) income.[33] This question needs further research but a recent investigation suggests that the "burden of dependency" (ratio of productive workers to total population) is an important explanation of the large differences in saving ratios among the countries of the world.[34] A representative sample of less developed countries with low dependency ratios shows that over 65 percent of total investment is devoted to maintaining the level of per capita income at a constant level, whereas the corresponding figure for a sample of developed countries (with high dependency ratios) was less than 25 percent.

Moreover, a cross-section study of 67 countries indicates that an increase of a little more than 1.5 percent points in the fraction of GNP invested is needed to offset the effects of a rise of one percentage point in the rate of population growth.[35]

Thirdly, if a reduction in fertility resulted in better nutritional and health status as well as increased education of the labor force, this would lead to a larger total income than otherwise due in part to improved labor quality. There are two reasons why nutrition and health would improve: First, the total population would be smaller, but total income and hence total expenditures on food consumption and health services might be larger. For both these reasons, each member of the labor force would be better nourished and healthier. Total expenditures on education might be greater, and after some time lag (the time between the start of the reduction in fertility and the age of entry to schools) the school age population would be smaller. Eventually, as a higher proportion of educated persons entered the labor force, the work force would become more highly skilled.

However, a reduction in fertility has an impact on the size of the labor force. Here it is important to make a distinction between the short term (defined as the time between birth and the average age at which persons enter the labor force, or about 15 years) and the long term. In the short run a reduction in fertility has no effect on the size of the labor force, since all the persons who will be entering the labor force over the next 15 years or so have already been born. In the long run there would be a negative effect since the work force will be smaller. However, if chronic widespread unemployment is a severe problem, a diminished rate of growth of the labor force could result in lower levels of joblessness with little actual effect on the national income.

Finally, a country with a substained high birth rate is forced to divert expenditures to those goods that have a high capital-output ratio such as educational and medical facilities. Thus, income tends to increase at a slower rate than is the case when a reduction in fertility permits a greater investment in projects with lower capital-output ratios such as agricultural or industrial enterprises.

Combining all of these effects, it is clear that a reduction in fertility can favorably affect the standard of living. On the one hand, there are fewer people; on the other, total output itself is larger in the short run under conditions of reduced fertility. After a period of 15 years, there is some doubt whether total income would be larger than otherwise since this depends on the relative magnitude of the several positive effects as compared to the negative effect of the smaller labor force.

In his work, *Asian Drama*, Gunnar Myrdal criticizes a number of assumptions underlying the Coale-Hoover model.[36] First, the authors assumed constancy in the capital-output ratio as well as certain institutional arrangements within India. If these assumptions were modified, the results might have been very different from those indicated above. One cannot realistically assume a constant capital-output ratio over a period of several decades. Myrdal also objects to the savings function adopted by Coale and Hoover, which implies that savings are a function of per capita income. First, Coale and Hoover exclude nonmonetary savings in India, an item which is actually of considerable importance. Furthermore, "the personal sector accounts for less than three-sevenths of total monetized savings, government for most of the rest, and corporations for a small but growing share."[37] Finally, since savings were assumed to be identified with capital accumulation, and capital accumulation is by assumption the only productive factor, the major contribution that population can make to total output is through its influence on the savings function.

Coale and Hoover also assume that the average propensity to save will double or triple between 1956 and 1986. This assumption of a growing savings rate for individuals conflicts with evidence in other countries including the United States. The assumption that government savings or corporate savings will vary directly with per capita income is equally questionable.[38] In general, Myrdal concludes that to be useful "models would have to contain many more parameters and account for many more interrelationships. They would have to be very much more complex in order to be logically consistent and correspond with reality. With the present dirth of empirical data, indulging in this type of preparatory macroanalysis data does not seem to be a rewarding endeavor."[39] This is thus not only a criticism of the Coale-Hoover model, but also of any relatively abstract, economic-demographic model in terms of its being a useful guide to policy.

The primary implication of the Coale-Hoover model is that rapid population growth inhibits economic development. Turning to an empirical study of this phenomena we should expect to find an inverse relationship between population growth and per capita income. That is, even if per capita income growth is in most cases positive, do those nations with low rates of growth of per capita income usually exhibit high population growth and do countries with high rates of economic growth have low rates of population growth? Table 6-2 summarizes the data for 37 less developed countries.

The statistics indicate little evidence of any significant association positive or negative between changes in income and rates of population growth. Thus, in some cases, high per capita income is associated with low population growth rates, and in some cases with high population growth rates. The same is true for countries with low per capita income. A similar study carried out by Simon Kuznets yielded the same conclusion. He studied 11 presently developed countries for which data were available for the half century prior to World War I.[40] Of course, in the comparison for the current period, if the recent experience of the presently developed countries were added, one would find that there was some indication that countries with higher growth rates of per capita income tended to have lower population growth rates. But if the less developed countries were added to the pre-World War I comparison, the reverse conclusion would obtain—those with higher per capita income growth rates tended to have higher population growth rates.[41]

None of the above discussion implies that per capita income growth would have been the same if population growth rates in any given country had been markedly higher or lower. However, the effect of population growth, whether positive or negative, is not so great relative to other growth determinants as to stand out in a simple comparison. This cautions against preoccupation with the effect of population growth on economic development to the exclusion of other determinants.

Table 6-2

Frequency Distribution of Developing Nations by Growth Rate of Real Per Capita Income, 1957-58 to 1963-64

Rate of Population Growth (Percent Per Year)	Total	Rate of Growth of Real Per Capita Income (Percent Per Year)						
		Less Than Zero	0 to 0.9	1.0 to 1.9	2.0 to 2.9	3.0 to 3.9	4.0 to 4.9	5.0 and Over
Total	37	3	4	12	12	2	2	2
3.5 and over	2	1	0	0	0	0	1	0
3.0-3.4	10	0	2	3	4	0	1	0
2.5-2.9	11	1	2	5	1	1	0	1
2.0-2.4	8	0	0	3	5	0	0	0
1.5-1.9	4	1	0	0	2	1	0	0
Less than 1.5	2	0	0	1	0	0	0	1

Source: Richard A. Easterlin, "Effects of Population Growth on the Economic Development of Developing Countries," in *The Annals of the American Academy of Political and Social Science*, Vol. 369, January 1967, p. 106.

Demographic Transition and Developing Countries

The process of change from a high mortality/high fertility to low mortality/high fertility and finally to low mortality/low fertility is known as the demographic transition. The causes of the mortality decline are factors such as improved health and sanitation practices and more efficient means of transportation and communication. Fertility declines have been associated with factors such as greater industrialization, compulsory schooling, and a recognition of the decline in infant mortality rates.

While the causes of fertility declines in developed countries are controversial, it is clear that the long-term trend has been downward throughout most of the twentieth century. By the 1970s fertility rates in nearly all developed countries had dropped to levels very close to "replacement."

The population history of the developing countries is very different. The decline in mortality began 40 to 50 years ago and has occurred much more rapidly than was the case in the developed countries. In large part the fall in mortality rates in developing countries has been unrelated to economic development but instead had been ascribed to the widespread adaption of relatively inexpensive public health measures including vaccination, eradication of disease bearing insects, and improved sanitation.

While birth rates have subsequently declined in many developing countries they have generally remained higher than in preindustrial Europe, while mortality declines have been dramatic. The result has been population growth rates in developing countries that average 2.5 percent per annum—a figure nearly 1.5 times greater than during Europe's most rapid period of population growth.[42]

There are two important reasons why birth rates in developing countries have only recently begun to slowly decline. First, the level of economic development and per capita income that was associated with declines in birth rates in developed countries will not be achieved in many countries in Asia and Africa for at least two generations. Until this "threshold of development" is reached one cannot expect the birth rate to fall because of economic progress. Secondly, birth rates remain high in developing countries because infant and child mortality rates remain high. There has been an increasing amount of research relating birth rates in developing countries to changes in infant and child mortality rates. Let us consider the findings of a number of the more important studies.

The Child Survival Hypothesiss

The decline in mortality of children under five has frequently been advanced as a major cause of a decrease in fertility rates.[43] The most commonly stated mechanism is that children are an economic asset to parents—a means for assuring them support in their old age as well as assisting in operating farms and other enterprises. Death of offspring contribute both directly and indirectly to fertility. If parents lose a child, they may replace that child through another birth. Moreover, the risk that children may die is responsible for a form of hedging on the part of parents. In communities where infant and child mortality rates are high, parents may increase the number of births they desire as a form of insurance against the eventuality of securing "too few" surviving children. As parents become more confident of the survival of their existing offspring, their need for additional children to ensure the minimum declines. Another mechanism underlying the observed mortality-fertility relationship is of biological origin. When an infant or young child dies, the mother ceases to lactate and the probability that she will conceive increases. It is not yet clear which of the two mechanisms is more important. In any case, government programs that promote reductions in mortality also tend to reduce fertility.

On the basis of a detailed survey by Alvin Harman in the Philippines, it appears that "replacement" due specifically to infant mortality is considerably greater than that due to child mortality. Moreover, fertility behavior is more closely associated with changes in the infant mortality rate in the community as a whole as compared to the number of infant deaths in the individual family.[44] Thus, the hedging by Philippine parents against loss of children seems to be an important consideration in predicting actual family size. As infant mortality is

Table 6-3

Average Number of Live Births and Expected Surviving Births for Turkish Women Under 45 Years of Age, by Socioeconomic Status, 1970

	Number of Live Births		Number of Expected Surviving Live Births[a]	
	With Experience of Infant Deaths	Without Experience of Infant Deaths	With Experience of Infant Deaths	Without Experience of Infant Deaths
Birthplace of parents				
Both urban	4.4	3.0	4.2	3.6
Mixed	4.4	3.2	4.2	4.1
Both village	5.6	4.4	5.0	5.4
Education of parents				
Both without school	5.8	4.5	5.2	5.3
One without and one with school; or both primary school only	5.0	3.7	4.7	4.8
One primary or above and one more than primary	3.7	2.8	3.2	3.1
Husband's monthly income				
< $70	5.3	3.9	4.8	4.8
$70-$139	4.8	3.3	4.3	3.9
> $140	3.9	2.6	3.1	3.0
Media exposure				
Low	5.6	4.2	5.0	5.1
Medium	4.8	3.4	4.2	3.9
High	3.7	2.7	3.1	3.1
Duration of marriage				
< 10 years	3.3	2.5	4.0	3.8
10-19 years	5.4	3.6	4.4	4.4
> 20 years	6.2	5.1	4.8	5.0

[a]Expected surviving births = surviving live births + additional expected live births.

Source: Carl E. Taylor, Jeanne S. Newman, and Narindar U. Kelly, "Health Aspects of Population Increase," Working Paper No. 8 for the World Population Conference, 1974, p. 19, processed.

reduced, families can be expected to have fewer replacement births and also to hedge to a lesser degree. Both of these changes will tend to offset the more rapid rate of natural increase that might otherwise result.

In Turkey when the number of live births is compared for women with and without infant deaths, the former have more children. (See Table 6-3.) This is true even when one standardizes for socioeconomic status. Similar results have been found in studies undertaken in Egypt[45] and Bangladesh.[46]

As one corollary of the child survival hypothesis, the time interval until the decline in fertility occurs may be expected to be shorter where rapid declines in infant mortality are or have been underway. Table 6-4 reports the distribution of the mean rate of fall in infant mortality and crude birth rates by the interval between the onset of decline in infant mortality (or 1945-49, whichever is later), and the apparent onset of fertility decline for 53 countries. Of these, in only one (Dominican Republic) was the post-World War II decline in infant mortality interrupted by a temporary rise after the onset of fertility decline. Among the other 52 countries, the shorter the interval between infant mortality and onset of fertility decline, the greater has been the mean postwar rate of fall in infant mortality, with a Spearman rank correlation coefficient of −1. For the 53 countries as a whole, the median interval to the onset of fertility decline, following 1945-49, or the subsequent onset of mortality decline, is only 11.4 years.[47] However, it is possible that the relationship is not causal; that it is not declining infant mortality that causes fertility decline, but that both are caused by other factors.

Recent evidence has indicated that in an increasing number of poor countries birth rates have fallen sharply in spite of relatively low per capita income and in spite of the absence or relative newness of family planning programs. The examination of these cases reveals a common factor. The countries in which this has happened are those in which the broadest spectrum of the population has shared in the economic and social benefits of significant national progress to a far greater degree than in most poor countries. (See Table 6-5.)

Table 6-4
Mean Rates of Decline in Infant Mortality Rate and Crude Birth Rate Since 1945-49 by Interval Between Decline in Infant Mortality and Onset of Decline in Crude Birth Rate

Interval Between Decline in IMR and CBR	Number of Countries	Rates of Change Since 1945-49 in:	
		Infant Mortality Rate	Crude Birth Rate
< 0 years	1[a]	−0.0361	−0.0178
< 5 years	6	−0.0496	−0.0219
5-9 years	16	−0.0373	−0.0165
10-14 years	14	−0.0353	−0.0238
15-19 years	13	−0.0327	−0.0146
> 20 years	3	−0.0288	−0.0000
Total	53	−0.0367	−0.0178

[a]Dominican Republic experienced a temporary rise in infant mortality after 1950-54, since reversed; crude birth rate has been declining since 1950-54, so that the birth rate fall appeared to precede the death rate fall even though in 1950-54 the CBR was 44.0 and the IMR was 79.7

Source: Carl E. Taylor, Jeanne S. Newman, and Narindar U. Kelly, "Health Aspects of Population Increase," Working Paper No. 8 for the World Population Conference, 1974, p. 15, processed.

Table 6-5
Comparison of the Economies of the Philippines, Taiwan, Mexico, Brazil and Korea

	Philippines	Taiwan	Mexico	Brazil	Korea
Per Capita income 1960:	$169	$176	$441	$268	$138
1969:	$208	$334	$606	$348	$242
GNP growth rates in 1960s	--	10%	7%	6%	9%
Annual increase in industrial jobs	--	10% (1963-69)	5.4% (1969-70)	2.8% (1966-69)	--
Unemployment and gross underemployment	14.5% (1961)	10% (1963)	Significant	--	--
	15% (1968)	4% (1968)	and rising	--	--
Ratio of income controlled by top 20% of income recipients to bottom 20%	12:1 (1956)	15:1 (1953)	10:1 (1950)	22:1 (1960)	5:1
	16:1 (1965)	5:1 (1969)	16:1 (1969)	25:1 (1970)	
Income improvement of poorest 20% over past 20 years	Negligible	200%	Negligible	Negligible	Over 100%
Investment cost of increasing GNP by $1 in 1960s	$3.50	$2.10	$3.10	$2.80	$1.70
Exports ($ millions) 1960:	$560	$164	$831	$1,269	$5.2
1970:	$961	$1,428	$1,402	$2,310	$835.2

Effective land reform	No	Yes	No	No	Yes
Agricultural working population per 100 hectares	71	195	35	43	197
Percentage of farmers belonging to cooperatives (late 1960s)	17%	Virtually 100%	5%	28%	Virtually 100%
Yields per acre for food grains	1,145 (1968-70)	3,570	1,225	1,280	2,850
Literacy	72%	85%	76%	67%	71%
Life expectancy	55	68	61	64	64
Infant mortality per 1,000 births	72	19	66	94	41
Rural households electrified	6%	75%	—	—	27%
Consumption of electric power (kilowatt hours per person)	39 (1951) 184 (1968)	116 (1949) 745 (1968)	162 (1948) 481 (1968)	200 (1952) 390 (1966)	55 (1953) 200 (1968)
Crude birth rates (births per thousand)	— 45 (1960) 44 (1970)	41 (1947) 36 (1963) 26 (1970)	44 (1950) 44 (1960) 41 (1970)	41 (1950) 41 (1960) 38 (1970)	45 (1950) 42 (1960) 30 (1970)

Source: William Rich, *Smaller Families Through Social and Economic Progress*, Monograph No. 7 (Washington, D.C.: Overseas Development Council, 1973), pp. 70-71.

Family planning programs generally have been more successful in those countries in which increases in output of goods and social services have been distributed in such a way that they improve the quality of life for a substantial majority of the population rather than just for a small minority.[48]

Thus, of the five countries, only in Taiwan and Korea has the distribution of income and social services become more equal and the birth rate fallen substantially. It appears that a more equal distribution of income and other developmental indices (due to a more rapid increase in the earnings of low income as compared to high income families), which is not only desirable in itself, is associated with a reduction in the rate of population growth.

Finally, as pointed out by Rich, the average income levels of the poorest 60 percent of the population correlate much more closely with fertility levels than do average incomes of the entire population. In a comparison of 40 less developed countries, an increase of $10 in the annual per capita income of the lower 60 percent was associated with a 0.7 per thousand decline in the crude birth rate, whereas a $10 increase in average income was associated with only a 0.3 per thousand decline.[49] These data provide further support for the hypothesis that the factor most crucial to fertility is increased distribution of income (and services) to the large low-income portion of the population.

Finally, there is an increasingly firm belief among some development experts that the goal of increasing per capita income has been overemphasized. These individuals stress the greater importance of *social* development and the important role that health programs can play in enhancing social development and the quality of life.

The quality of life should be an important element in the goals of development in all cultural contexts.[50] However, in a practical sense, one must define the terms "social development" or "quality of life" in order that they have operational or policy significance. Thus, "we have measures of death and illness, but no measures of physical vigor or mental health. We have measures of the level and distribution of income, but no measures of the satisfaction that income brings. We have measures of air and water pollution, but no way to tell whether an environment is on balance, becoming uglier, or more beautiful. We have some clues about the test performance of children, but no information about their creativity or attitude toward intellectual endeavor."[51]

However, the importance of social development, even if measurable, can also be overemphasized. Many nations have desperately low levels of income. The income gap between rich and poor nations is widening. If the goal of economic growth and progress in developing nations is sidetracked, could not the developed countries and their economic experts be accused of "copping out" by redefining the goal to be that of social development? Clearly both economic development and social development are important. Each society will have to determine the relative importance of each in terms of its own aspirations.

Summary

Health programs can increase the rate of economic progress by (1) increasing the quality of the labor force, (2) allowing new regions to be settled and developed, or old regions redeveloped, and (3) engendering new attitudes toward entrepreneurship and new initiatives. Regarding the latter, Wilfred Malenbaum's work is an important first step in quantifying the importance of health on attitude changes and subsequent development.

The Coale-Hoover model implies strongly that rapid population growth inhibits an increase in per capita income. However, the empirical work of Richard Easterlin and Simon Kuznets does not support the implications of the Coale-Hoover model. Moreover, Gunnar Myrdal provides several important criticisms of the underlying assumptions of the model.

Birth rates have begun to fall in a large number of developing countries. Recent work by Carl E. Taylor and his colleagues indicates that this fall is preceded by a decline in the infant mortality rate. This tends to confirm the validity of the child survival hypothesis. In addition, the evidence suggests that acceptance of family-planning programs and declines in national birth rates are affected by the distribution of income and availability of social services.

Notes

1. Harold Frederiksen, "Determinants and Consequences of Mortality Trends in Ceylon," *Public Health Reports*, Vol. 76, 1961, p. 660.

2. Peter Newman, *Malaria Eradication and Population Growth with Special Reference to Ceylon and British Guiana* (Ann Arbor, Michigan: Bureau of Public Health Economics, 1965), pp. 67-69.

3. Carl E. Taylor and Marie-Francoise Hall, "Health Population and Economic Development," *Science*, Vol. 157, August 1967, p. 3.

4. Charles Winslow, *The Cost of Sickness and the Price of Health* (Geneva, Switzerland: World Health Organization, 1951), p. 22.

5. Winslow, *The Cost of Sickness*, p. 25.

6. Ibid., p. 30.

7. B.A. Weisbrod, R.L. Andreano, R.E. Baldwin, E.H. Epstein, and A.C. Kelley, "Disease and Economic Development: The Impact of Parasitic Diseases in St. Lucia," unpublished manuscript, February 1971, pp. 111-245.

8. H.A. Kraut and E.A. Muller, "Calorie Intake and Industrial Output," *Science*, Vol. 104, November 1946, p. 495.

9. Winslow, *The Cost of Sickness*, p. 33.

10. Taylor and Hall, *Health Population*, p. 3.

11. Selma Mushkin, *International Development Review*, Vol. 6, 1964, p. 10.

12. Taylor and Hall, *Health Population*, p. 3.

13. Paul Enterline and William Stewart, "Health Improvements, Worker Productivity, and Levels of Living in Rapidly Growing Countries," paper presented before the American Academy of Arts and Sciences, 1960.

14. Wilfred Malenbaum, "Health and Expansion in Poor Lands," *International Journal of Health Services*, Vol. 3, No. 2, Spring, 1973, p. 169.

15. Helen Nash, "Life Blooms in the Rapti Valley," *War on Hunger: A Report from the Agency for International Development*, Vol. 8, No. 10, October, 1974, pp. 11-12.

16. World Health Organization, "The Economic Benefits of Malaria Eradication," unpublished, 1957, p. 3.

17. John M. Hunter, "River Blindness in Nangodi, Northern Ghana: A Hypothesis of Cyclical Advance and Retreat," *The Geographical Review*, Vol. 56, July 1966, No. 3, pp. 409-10.

18. Hunter, "River Blindness," pp. 415-16.

19. J.M.D. Roberts, "The Control of Epidemic Malaria in the Highlands of Western Kenya," *Journal of Tropical Medicine and Hygiene*, Vol. 67, September 1964, pp. 230-37.

20. Norman Holly, "Economic Benefits of Malaria Control in Ethiopia," unpublished paper, Agency for International Development, 1970.

21. Peter A. Ruderman, comment on "Some Economic Aspects of Public Health Programs in Underdeveloped Areas," in *Economics of Health and Medical Care* (Ann Arbor, Michigan: University of Michigan, 1964), pp. 299-305.

22. Malenbaum, "Health and Expansion," pp. 169-70.

23. Joaquin Craviato and Elsa R. DeLicardie, "The Effect of Malnutrition on the Individual," and J.M. Bengoa, "Significance of Malnutrition and Priorities for Its Prevention," and Alan Berg, Nevin Scrimshaw and David Call (Eds.), *Nutrition, National Development and Planning* (Cambridge, Massachusetts: MIT Press, 1973), pp. 3-21 and pp. 103-28.

24. Wilfred Malenbaum, "Health and Productivity in Poor Areas," in Herbert E. Klarman (Ed.), *Empirical Studies in Health Economics* (Baltimore, Maryland: The Johns Hopkins Press, 1970), p. 38.

25. Malenbaum, "Health and Productivity," p. 49.

26. Weisbrod, et al., "Disease and Economic Development," p. 41.

27. Ibid., p. 44.

28. Association of American Medical Colleges, *The Population Problem* (Evanston, Illinois: Association of American Medical Colleges, 1970), p. 3.

29. Warren Robinson and David Horlacher, "Population Growth and Economic Welfare," *Reports on Population/Family Planning*, No. 6, The Population Council, February 1971, p. 10.

30. A.J. Coale and E.M. Hoover, *Population Growth and Economic Development in Low Income Countries: A Case Study of India's Prospects* (Princeton, New Jersey: Princeton University Press, 1958), p. 261. For a complete description of the model, see pp. 282-83.

31. Robinson and Horlacher, "Population Growth," p. 11.

32. Coale and Hoover, "Population Growth," p. 271.

33. George C. Zaidan, "Population Growth and Economic Development," *Finance and Development*, Vol. 6, No. 3, September 1969, p. 3.

34. N.H. Luff, "Population Growth and Savings Potential," unpublished preliminary report of the Office of Program Coordination, U.S. Agency for International Development, 1969.

35. Paul M. Sommers and Daniel S. Suits, "A Cross-Section Model of Economic Growth," *The Review of Economics and Statistics*, Vol. 53, No. 2, May 1971, pp. 121-28.

36. Gunnar Myrdal, *Asian Drama—An Inquiry into the Poverty of Nations* (New York: Random House, 1968), Appendix 7, pp. 2068-75.

37. Myrdal, *Asian Drama*, p. 2073.

38. Robinson and Horlacher, "Population Growth," p. 13.

39. Myrdal, *Asian Drama*, p. 2075.

40. Simon Kuznets, "Quantitative Aspects of the Economic Growth of Nations," Part I: "Levels and Variability of Rates of Growth," *Economic Development and Cultural Change*, Vol. 5, No. 1, October 1956, p. 30.

41. Jean Bourgeois-Pichat, "Population Growth and Development," *International Conciliation*, No. 556, January 1966, p. 15.

42. Michael S. Teitelbaum, "Population and Development: Is a Consensus Possible?" *Foreign Affairs*, Vol. 52, No. 4, July 1974, pp. 745-46.

43. See for example, Irma Adelman, "An Econometric Analysis of Population Growth," *American Economic Review*, Vol. 53, No. 3, pp. 314-39; Alvin Harman, *Fertility and Economic Behavior of Families in the Philippines* (Santa Monica: The Rand Corporation, RM-6385-AID, September 1970); and Mark Nerlove, T.P. Schultz, *Love and Life Between the Censuses: A Model of Family Decision Making in Puerto Rico, 1950-1960* (Santa Monica: The Rand Corporation, RM-6322-AID, September 1970).

44. Harman, *Fertility*, p. 37.

45. S.H. Hassan, "Influence of Child Mortality on Fertility," paper presented at the annual meeting of the Population Association of America, April 1966.

46. T. Paul Schultz and Julie DaVanzo, *Analysis of Demographic Change in East Pakistan: A Study of Retrospective Survey Data* (Santa Monica: The Rand Corporation, R-564-AID, September 1970), pp. 32-35.

47. Carl E. Taylor, Jeanne S. Newman, and Narindar U. Kelly, "Health Aspects of Population Increase," Working Paper No. 8, for the World Population Conference, 1974, processed, pp. 6-7.

48. Peter Adamson, "A Population Policy and a Development Policy Are One and the Same Thing," *The New Internationalist*, No. 15, May 1974, p. 9.

49. William Rich, *Smaller Families Through Social and Economic Progress*, Monograph No. 7 (Washington, D.C.: Overseas Development Council, 1973), pp. 15-16.

50. Abraham Horwitz, "Summary of Human Values Workshop," paper presented at International Health Conference, April 27, 1973, pp. 31-32.

51. Wilbur J. Cohen, *Toward A Social Report* (Washington, D.C.: U.S. Government Printing Office, 1969), p. XIV. For a pioneering effort to measure the quality of life see: A.D. Charnes, W.W. Cooper, and G. Kozmetsky, "Measuring, Monitoring and Modeling Quality of Life," *Management Science*, Vol. 19, No. 10, June 1973, p. 1172.

7

Health and Poverty

This chapter focuses on the interrelationship between low income and health status. The association between income and mortality, and morbidity and utilization of health services are explored. Health programs for the poor including the Neighborhood Center and Medicaid will be examined. Finally, an evaluation will be made of the health program operated by the Public Health Service for American Indians residing on reservations.

Health Status and Poverty

The precise meaning of the term "poverty" is difficult to determine because some type of value judgment is required to specify a poverty level of income. The definition of poverty level of income may be expressed in either relative or absolute terms. A relativistic approach to the definition of poverty could, for example, indicate that all those individuals in the lower 25 percent of the income distribution receive poverty level incomes.

However, most of the poverty statistics used by government agencies are based on a so-called "poverty-index" that was developed by the Social Security Administration in 1964. For families of three or more persons, the poverty level was set at three times the cost of an economy food plan developed by the U.S. Department of Agriculture to provide minimum nutritional needs for "emergency or temporary use when funds are low." Annual revisions of the poverty-income cutoff, which in 1964 was $3,000 for a family of four, were formerly based upon price changes for the items in the economy food budget. Since 1969 the poverty-income levels have been revised upward to reflect similar movements in the overall consumer price index.[1] In 1971 the low income or poverty threshold—the income level that separates "poor" from "nonpoor"—was $4,137 for a nonfarm family of four.[2]

There are wide variations in the incidence of poverty among the various subgroups of the population. Thus, the likelihood that a family headed by a woman will have an income below the poverty level is five times greater than a family with a male head. Roughly 1 in 10 whites is below the poverty-income level, compared with one-third of all blacks. Thus, while only 11 percent of the population is black, this group accounted for nearly three-tenths of all persons classified as poor in 1971. Families living on farms are twice as likely to be below the poverty-income level as those living elsewhere and those family heads with an elementary school education were four-times more likely to earn incomes below the poverty level as high school graduates.

The supply of health services is finite and therefore available only in limited degree to the entire population. Thus, health may be considered, in economic terms, a scarce good. In most societies, whatever the prevailing system of social stratification, the scarce goods of life are likely to be distributed unequally. This is especially true when the service is provided by private individuals on a fee-for-service basis. Thus, there exists a strong association between poverty and ill health.

Income and Mortality

Major problems exist in the use of mortality data to measure the impact of income on health. If family income is used as the explanatory variable, it is likely that in some cases the family income has been reduced prior to death because of illness. In all cases it is difficult to obtain reliable information for individuals since death certificates do not classify individuals according to socioeconomic status.[3] Thus, a number of studies have related death rates for geographic units to selected characteristics of the population in the areas. For example, Monroe Lerner compares death rates (including infant mortality rates) for poverty and nonpoverty areas of Chicago. The age-adjusted death rates were 40 percent higher in the poverty areas.[4] Moreover, the infant mortality rate in the poverty areas was nearly double the rate in all other areas. A study of death rates by counties in California for different age groups produced striking results. As expected, income was negatively related to the death rate as was surprisingly enough, the proportion Spanish in each county, while the percentage black and a pesticide use index were positively related to the death rate.[5]

The National Center for Health Statistics collected data on reported deaths in 1962-63. Questionnaires were sent to the families to obtain socioeconomic data relevant to the deceased person and his family. Harold Luft used this data to develop information relating death rates and family income. (See Table 7-1.)

As indicated above, there are substantial differences by income class. First the gradient relating to death rates and income levels is greatest for males in the prime working ages. This would be expected if there were an important line of causation from low income to high mortality.[6] However, it is likely that many of the younger men die after a certain period of illness, which reduces their family income. It would then be expected that more deaths would occur in low-income families than would be the case if a more permanent measure of income were used. Second, the death rate differences are somewhat smaller for women (which supports the hypothesis that some of those in the lower income classes are there because of poor health). However, the differences are still substantial. Third, those under 25, whose family income should be least sensitive

Table 7-1

Deaths Per 10,000 Population by Age, Sex, and Family Income, United States, 1962-63

Age at Death	Family Income in Year Before Death					(1)/(5)
	$2,000	$2,000-$3,999	$4,000-$5,999	$6,000-$7,999	$8,000 +	
	(1)	(2)	(3)	(4)	(5)	
Males						
< 25	58	28	26	18	10	5.8
25-44	147	54	23	17	15	9.8
45-54	350	163	100	60	43	8.1
55-64	492	276	195	164	106	4.6
65 and over	776	672	623	494	349	2.2
Females						
< 25	41	19	17	9	5	8.2
25-44	64	21	15	9	9	7.1
45-54	132	54	62	27	21	6.3
55-64	194	109	101	63	53	3.6
65 and over	411	395	464	436	345	1.2

Source: Harold Luft, *Poverty and Health: An Empirical Investigation of the Economic Interactions*, unpublished doctoral dissertation, Harvard University, 1972, p. 78.

to the impact of their illness, still exhibit great discrepancies in death rates. Thus, even when adjustments are made to remove the adverse effects of health on income, there is a substantial impact of income on death rates.[7]

Income and Morbidity

Measurement of illness for large populations has typically been accomplished through health surveys. One of the prime sources of health survey data is the National Center for Health Statistics. The center conducts intensive interviews with a sample of 42,000 households each year obtaining health status and utilization information on about 135,000 persons.[8]

Differences in the frequency of acute conditions by income levels are very small. For example, the incidence of all acute conditions per hundred persons per year for the period July 1962 to June 1963, age-adjusted, for the income categories under $2,000, $2,000 to $3,999, $4,000 to $6,999, and $7,000 and over, were 216, 204, 216, and 232 respectively.[9] By definition, all acute conditions included in these rates either were attended medically or caused at least one day of restricted activity. Thus, these rates combine the effects of an underlying illness and the individual's response to that illness.

Turning to chronic conditions, a clearer picture emerges with respect to the relationship between this type of illness and income. This may be seen in Table 7-2. For each age category, the proportion of the lowest income group with one or more activity limiting chronic conditions is greater than any of the higher income groups.

In addition, for a number of particular chronic conditions there is a definite pattern of higher prevalence as the income level decreases. On a rate basis per 1,000 population, those with less than $2,000 family income report more than four times as many heart conditions as those in the highest income group; six times as much mental and nervous trouble; six times as much arthritis and rheumatism; six times as many cases of high blood pressure; over three times as many orthopedic impairments (excluding paralysis and absence of limbs); and almost eight times as many visual impairments.[10]

Luft has reviewed a large number of studies relating activity limitation and economic status. "Although certainly some of the observed differences are due to the effects of poor health, resulting in a loss of income or a change in occupation, a large fraction of the observed relationship is due to the effects of income-education-occupation on health."[11]

Utilization and Income

A number of studies have indicated a strong positive correlation between physician and dental visits per year and family income.[12] However, *recent* data suggest that there is little correlation between average number of physician visits per year and family income. Based on information gathered from household interviews in 1969, the average number of physician visits was 4.8 per persons in families with less than $3,000 income, and 4.3 for persons whose income was over $10,000.[13] But these averages mask a strong relationship for children under 15 years of age. For those whose family income is under $3,000, the average number of physician visits from July 1966 to June 1967 was 4.4 for children under 5, and 1.5 for those 5 to 14 years of age; for those whose family income is over $10,000, the average for the corresponding ages were 7.2 and 3.5.[14] Taking education of the head of the family into account, however, the correlation between family income and average annual number of physician visits among children disappears. (See Table 7-3.) These statistics imply that education of parents is more important than income in determining physician visits for children.

Moreover, information collected by the National Center for Health Statistics indicates that while income is related specifically to the utilization of medical specialists, education seems more strongly related in general to utilization than income.

These results imply that health-related and health-oriented behavior is partly

Table 7-2

Percent of Population with Chronic Conditions Causing Activity Limitation by Age and Family Income, United States, July 1965-June 1966

		Family Income				
	All Incomes	Under $3,000	$3,000-$4,999	$5,000-$6,999	$7,000-$9,999	$10,000 +
All ages	11.2	25.4	12.1	7.9	6.9	6.8
Under 17 years	1.9	2.6	1.6	1.5	1.6	1.7
17-44	7.3	13.1	8.6	6.4	5.8	5.4
45-64	18.9	38.5	22.5	15.9	13.8	10.4
65 and over	45.1	50.6	42.4	42.1	38.8	38.6

Source: National Center for Health Statistics, *Limitations on Activity and Mobility Due to Chronic Conditions, United States, July 1965-June 1966*, Series 10, No. 45 (Washington, D.C.: U.S. Government Printing Office, 1968), p. 29.

Table 7-3

Number of Physician Visits Per Person Per Year by Education of Head of Family and Family Income for Persons Under 15 Years of Age, July 1966-June 1967

Family Income	Under 5 Years	5-8 Years	9-12 Years	13 + Years
Under $5,000	2.1	2.2	3.2	5.4
$5,000 and over	1.4	2.6	4.1	5.0

Source: National Center for Health Statistics, *Volume of Physician Visits, 1966-1967,* Series 10, No. 49 (Washington, D.C.: U.S. Government Printing Office, 1968), p. 19.

a matter of preference and that education is a primary agent in the development of such preferences. Moreover, the more educated a person, the more likely he is to have the opportunity to be exposed to and to be influenced by health information. His opportunities are greater because the media to which he is exposed is more likely to provide that information.[15]

Thomas Bice, Robert Eichhorn, and Peter Fox have shown that over the last 40 years, the relationship between family income and physician use has diminished substantially.[16] There has been a relative increase in the utilization of physicians by the poor and a relative decrease in use by the nonpoor. Medicare and Medicaid have probably played a major role in increasing demand for physician services among the poor. This interpretation is supported by findings from studies showing that physician use among low-income groups is particularly sensitive to the out-of-pocket costs they must pay. Moreover, the distribution of education, having become more equal, has resulted in a more equitable distribution of physician utilization.

However, while it is encouraging to note that the utilization of physicians by the poor is becoming more similar to that of the nonpoor, this finding should not make one complacent. It has been shown that low-income persons have more periods of illness than other individuals. Thus, truly equal access to health care would imply a *greater* utilization of physicians by low-income persons in comparison with others.

From multivariate analyses of data from a 1963 nationwide survey, Ronald Andersen and Lee Benham conclude that

Lower income groups seem particularly sensitive to the method of financing. Insurance coverage for the low-income groups apparently results in a dramatic increase in the demand for medical services. This fall in price to the consumer of medical care diminishes the importance of income as a determinant of the consumption of medical care.[17]

Other studies support this assertion; W.C. Richardson's studies of three OEO target areas show that the availability of third-party coverage reduced income differences in patient-initiated physician use.[18] Bice found that the poor in the

Baltimore metropolitan area, with Medicaid coverage, were more likely than the poor with no insurance coverage to visit physicians within a year.[19]

Poor Health as a Cause of Low Income

There is substantial evidence that many persons live at poverty-level incomes *because of poor health.* For instance, among men between the ages of 25 and 59, not in the labor force in March 1968, 51.9 percent of the whites and 62.9 percent of the blacks list health as the cause.[20] Even if the men are in the labor force, their health status will affect their vulnerability to unemployment. Data obtained by Herbert S. Parnes indicates that among white men whose health limited the amount or kind of work they could undertake, their unemployment rate was 140 percent higher than for those white males with no health limitations. The unemployment differences for blacks (with health limitations as compared to without) was 90 percent.[21] Luft found, using 1959 data, that the average loss of earnings to a spending unit head was $1,340, or about 31 percent of the $4,324 average annual earnings of the nondisabled head.[22]

The effects of disability can also be evaluated by considering the proportion of families with poverty level incomes. A crude estimate is that of the total number of husband-wife families with the head under 65 years in 1965 in poverty was 3.2 million. Disabled "families" account for about 77 percent of the poor nonaged husband-wife families in the United States.[23] This is not to say that this proportion of poverty is *due* to illness but that the income effects of poor health are substantial.

A number of studies have documented the decline in income that occurs after one becomes ill. For example, a study based on a sample of Social Security disability applicants in New Orelans, Minneapolis-St. Paul, and the Columbus, Ohio, areas who were not institutionalized indicated that median income fell from $482 to $220 per month after disability.[24] An earlier investigation concerned a 20 year follow-up survey of Hagerstown, Maryland, families. No families suffered a reduction in socioeconomic status if they were well at the beginning and end of the period, while 9.2 percent of the families that had an illness in 1943, after being free of illness in 1923, had a reduction in socioeconomic status.[25]

Neighborhood Health Centers

The amount and quality of health care received by the poor before the establishment of Neighborhood Health Centers was totally inadequate. "Care to the poor is typified by dismal settings—long waits, hard benches, and crowded waiting rooms; a lengthy series of eligibility screening interviews; insensitive treatment by hurried professionals; and a total lack of continuity. The result is care of the lowest quality—entirely fragmented and presented without regard to language and cultural differences or to human dignity."[26] One of the most fundamental problems has been access to any type of medical care. In Denver, for example, some patients now served by two Neighborhood Health Centers, previously were required to travel for over an hour to Denver General Hospital on a bus route that cost 60 cents. Moreover, no service was available on evenings and weekends. Patients from Columbia Point in Boston had to travel 90 minutes by bus and subway in order to reach the nearest free clinic. In East Palo Alto, California, prior to the establishment of the Neighborhood Health Center there were no dentists and only two physicians serving an area of 28,000 persons.[27]

The congressional mandate in November 1966 establishing the OEO Comprehensive Health Services Program was quite broad: ". . . to assure that (health) services are made readily accessible to residents of such areas (of concentrated poverty), are furnished in a manner most responsive to their needs and with their participation and whenever possible are combined with . . . arrangements for providing employment, education, social or other assistance needed by the families and individuals served. . . ."[28] Thus, two concepts became an integral part of all OEO health programs: (1) training community residents in new jobs as health workers and to be agents for community change; and (2) community involvement in planning and conducting the program.

Between 1965 and 1974, about 120 Neighborhood Health Centers and other comprehensive health service projects were initiated with OEO grant assistance. When the responsibility for OEO activities was transferred to other agencies, HEW took responsibility for funding Neighborhood Health Centers. Over $600 million has been invested in these efforts. This undertaking has been the largest governmental effort in the history of the United States to expand ambulatory health care resources in poor communities. It is estimated that Neighborhood Health Centers are serving a minimum of three million persons.[29]

A wide variety of health care agencies have joined in operating Neighborhood Health Centers. Community and teaching hospitals, medical schools, health departments, and individuals providing care in a group practice setting have been willing to assume these new or broader responsibilities. (See Table 7-4.)

Community Participation

The principle that consumers should participate actively in the development of policies for the centers was a key feature of the original concept of the Neighborhood Health Center and has been a major part of its operation.

The initial projects were generally developed by the professional staffs of health agencies who were primarily interested in improving the methods of

Table 7-4
Administering Agencies of Neighborhood Health Centers, 1965-71

Type of Administering Agency	Number of Projects
New Health Corporation	30
Hospital	16
Medical school	14
Health department	7
Group practice	7
Other	7
Total	81

Source: Daniel I. Zwick, "Some Accomplishments and Findings of Neighborhood Health Centers," *Milbank Memorial Fund Quarterly*, Vol. 50, October 1972, p. 393.

delivering health services to the poor. The participation of consumers has increased steadily, often resulting in a modification of the health center's organization. By participating on advisory and governing boards, consumers have played an important role in the development of almost all centers. Their specific activities have most often related to the selection of key staff, service priorities, hours of service, budgets, recruitment of outreach workers, and other local personnel and grievances.[30]

A study by Gerald Sparer, George Dines and Daniel Smith of 26 centers visited from 1967 to 1969 rated 7 centers high in the degree of consumer involvement, 9 moderate, and 10 low.[31] No pattern was apparent that would relate the type of administering agency to the degree of involvement. However, a positive relationship was found between outstanding personalities and consumer group involvement. Moreover, a strong staff personality oriented towards providers tended to limit consumer group involvement.

Consumer "demands" for health services in Neighborhood Health Centers have not been unlike those of other consumers. Generally, interest has focused on the need for more comprehensive services including dental care and drug abuse control services as well as additional hours of service. The desire for broader benefits parallels those indicated by consumers participating in prepaid group practices.[32]

Families usually "register" for care at the Neighborhood Health Centers (NHCs). They have not been required to make the center their sole or prime source of health care. However, this policy makes it difficult to achieve continuity of care. For example, an OEO-sponsored evaluation found that 72 percent of the user families considered the health center their "usual source of care" with a range of 48 to 91 percent.[33] Moreover, even among those indicating the center as their "usual source," about one-fourth of the participants stated their last physician visit was elsewhere. Similar results are found with respect to dental visits. Finally, nearly two-fifths of those surveyed indicated that they go to another source for the treatment of their most limiting condition.

The quality of care at the health centers has been found to compare favorably with other providers. Thus, a study by Gerald Sparer and Joyce Johnson of 33 NHCs indicated that 22 of 33 centers received the highest rating possible in terms of comprehensiveness of care,[34] and that two-thirds of the evaluated health centers offered care superior to that of nearby hospital outpatient departments.

A study of the utilization of services at eight health centers has indicated that enrollees average 4 to 5 doctor visits a year.[35] Surprisingly enough, even with complete removal of financial barriers and extensive outreach efforts and transportation services, the use of health care services by poor families did not rise markedly. However, the ability of health centers to reduce the need for costly inpatient care has been documented. For example, a study at the Mile Square Health Center in Chicago indicates the annual rate of inpatient days per 1,000 was reduced from about 1,000 to about 750 over three years. Even lower rates of inpatient care have been reported from projects in Boston and Portland, Oregon.

Approximately 1,000 physicians are currently employed in health centers, with about two-fifths on a full-time basis. The turnover rate appears to be relatively high with a "half life" of about two years.[36]

The employment of outreach staffs usually called "family health workers" or "community health aides" has been the method by which the centers have tried to improve utilization of services. Since over half the staff of the centers are residents of poverty neighborhoods these centers do have a positive employment effect. However, as indicated above, these individuals have not made an impact on utilization rates. A greater effort must be made to change the attitudes of the poor regarding the importance of modern medical care.

Costs and Financing

The initial OEO grant support of health centers assumed that long-term financial support would come from Medicare, Medicaid, and other financing sources. Thus, it was expected that funds from Medicaid and Medicare might finance 70 to 80 percent of health center costs.

However, the way in which the Medicaid program has evolved has prevented the achievement of this goal. State programs have been restrictive in terms of both beneficiary eligibility and supported services. As pointed out by Daniel I. Zwick, "Even the most successful efforts by health centers to obtain Medicaid, Medicare and other private third-party funds has resulted in reimbursements for only 50 percent or so of their budgets; in most cases, such payments have been in the range of 10-20 percent."[37]

Problems have also been experienced by health centers in obtaining payments under Medicare. Different policies have been applied to centers administered by hospitals and to "physician-directed clinics." Both Medicare and Medicaid have tended to treat hospital sponsored projects more liberally with regard to reimbursement.

Sparer and Johnson found that NHCs have provided clinical services at costs comparable to that of private providers. Annual per capita costs are competitive with those reported for major prepayment group practices as well as hospital outpatient departments. The cost of supporting services unique to NHC operations are less than 20 percent of total cost and often are less than 10 percent.[38]

The annual per capita costs attributable to outreach, transportation, and such special items as in-service education, are less than the cost of a half-day of inpatient care. If health centers can continue to achieve significant savings in the use of inpatient care they will be in a strong position to finance such services on a long-term basis.

Medicaid

Medicaid is a federal-state program with substantial federal participation. No state is required to have a Medicaid program, but if it does not, the federal financial support for medical care costs of a substantial proportion of its population is not available.

Medicaid is the largest public program specifically directed at providing services to the poor and the medically indigent. It is not one program but 52 with differing coverage and separate state administrators.[a] Medicaid reached more than one-third of the poor and medically indigent in 1971 when the program served about 13 million people.[39] Medicare, on the other hand, has removed much of the burden of acute-health care expenses for nearly all elderly persons. It provides medical insurance coverage (primarily hospital insurance) to over 95 percent of the aged. Nonetheless, in recent years Medicare has covered slightly less than half of the health-care expenditures of the aged. The out-of-pocket expenses are not only the deductibles and co-insurance, but also include drugs and the expenses associated with long-term care. Medicaid provides supplementary aid not only to the aged but also to other "categorical" groups, including children. It is significant that of the total Medicaid budget about 45 percent goes to the elderly, principally to cover the gaps that arise because Medicare covers only half their health-care expenditures. In addition, approximately 47 percent of the aged avail themselves of supplementary benefits from private carriers that significantly extend the protection of Medicare.

As in the case with other public assistance provisions of the Social Security

[a]Forty-eight states plus the District of Columbia, Guam, Puerto Rico, and the Virgin Islands have programs. Neither Arizona nor Alaska has a Medicaid program.

Act, no specific and detailed rules and standards were initially established by the federal government as to the eligibility conditions that may be required of applicants. Instead the states were required to determine the limits of income and resources in order to meet the condition that federal financial assistance be given only to persons "whose income and resources are insufficient to meet the costs of necessary medical services."

The 1967 Amendments to the Social Security Act, however, established an upper limit on net income, after deduction for medical expenses, for persons to whom federal matching funds under Medicaid would be made available. This limit was set at 133 1/3 percent of the cash-assistance standard actually being paid under the state's Aid to Families with Dependent Children Program for a family of comparable size.[40]

States can include in the Medicaid program those who are in the categorical public assistance groups, but who are not in financial need other than for their medical care costs. Typically, this would include individuals who are able to get along in normal circumstances, but who have heavy or unusual medical expenses at some time. This category may be termed the medically needy or indigent (as contrasted with cash-assistance recipients).

These regulations have produced wide variations among the states in the generosity of eligibility standards and benefit levels. Only half of the states provide coverage for the medically indigent, and the income cutoff point for a medically indigent family of four ranges from $2,500 in Oklahoma to $6,000 in New York.[41] Thus, nearly poor families may have most medical expenses paid if they live in one state and be completely unprotected if they live in another.

Bruce C. Stuart and Lee A. Bair examined the impact of the Medicaid and Medicare programs on the distribution of income. In 1966-67, for example, Medicaid recipients received an average of $33 in benefits for each dollar of costs, while Medicare recipients obtained only $3.35 in benefits per dollar of contributions. An average Medicaid household netted $852 worth of services for the year, while the net gain to Medicare households averaged $197.[42] Thus, as a redistributive measure Medicaid was considerably more effective than Medicare.

Since July 1969 Medicaid recipients have had free choice of qualified medical facilities, physicians, and pharmacies. Before then the state plan could restrict medical services to facilities and doctors who agreed to participate and were on a register established by the state.

By 1969 the total cost of the Medicaid program had reached nearly $4 billion, with the cost split almost evenly between the federal government and the states. The cost of the program rose more rapidly than the federal government had anticipated. The two major factors were the greater utilization of services than expected and the rapid rise in medical care costs. Only four years later costs had reached nearly $9 billion.[43]

Payments under Medicaid, the second largest federal health program, were about 15 percent higher in 1973 than in the previous year. A substantial portion of this increased cost resulted from payments to intermediate care facilities. For the first time a full year of payments for intermediate care facilities appeared as a reimbursable item under Medicaid. Before January 1972 payments for this type of service were made by cash-assistance programs. Intermediate care facilities provide institutional health services to persons who require more than custodial care but less intensive care than that provided by a hospital or skilled nursing facility. Nearly one-third of Medicaid's 1973 outlays were spent for intermediate care facilities and nursing home care—both less expensive alternatives than hospitalization.[44]

Medicaid and Utilization of Health Services

The effect of Medicaid on the utilization of health services is unclear. The studies reviewed in this section offer conflicting results.

A study of low-income persons in New York City indicated that Medicaid did result in some shift in the location or type of care received. (See Table 7-5.)

By 1970 nearly 12 times as many individuals were receiving their primary source of care from a private doctor and nearly 25 percent fewer had no main place of care. However, the majority of persons did not alter the location of their source of health services. The primary reason was that even though financial barriers were removed, many preferred other alternatives to using a private physician. Among those that preferred a private doctor but continued to use a clinic or emergency room, such factors as distance, hours of service, need for specialized facilities and physician refusal to accept Medicaid patients were the most important considerations.[45]

In Boston the Medicaid program has had a major impact on utilization of dental services by low-income persons. Within a year after the program went into

Table 7-5
Reported Main Place for Medical Care, Full Follow-up Residents

	1963-64	1969-70
Private doctor	7 (1.0%)	82 (11.7%)
City hospital	232 (32.2%)	225 (32.1%)
Voluntary hospital	288 (40.1%)	274 (39.0%)
Other or unspecified place	60 (8.4%)	24 (3.4%)
No main place	131 (18.2%)	97 (13.8%)
Total	718 (100.0%)	702 (100.0%)

Source: Margaret C. Olendzki, Richard P. Grann, and Charles H. Goodrich, "The Impact of Medicaid on Private Care for the Urban Poor," *Medical Care*, May-June 1972, Vol. 10, No. 3, p. 202.

effect, the percentage of respondents reporting a regular source of dental care rose from 64 percent to 76 percent; and the percentage of respondents who went to private practitioners increased from 37 percent to 58 percent. Moreover, the proportion of clinic users fell from 27 percent to 19 percent.[46]

A study in Chicago examining Medicaid utilization patterns showed that substantial numbers of Medicaid patients bypass nearby community hospitals and receive care in more distant teaching hospitals. In addition to possible negative medical consequences, the pattern is much more expensive to the state's Medicaid program than care in closer community hospitals would be.

It is likely that the following factors account for this phenomenon:

1. *Uncertainty about eligibility status.* At the time of admission a prospective patient must prove that he can pay for care. Some people are not able to do this when admitted even though they may be eligible for Medicaid benefits. This is especially true of the people who do not receive cash assistance, but whose incomes are sufficiently low to place them in the medically indigent category. The hospital takes a risk if it admits them since they might not subsequently be judged eligible.

2. *The absence of a personal physician with hospital privileges.* The presumption may be that the doctor has enough contact with the patient to know whether or not he can pay for services. Moreover, even if a person could demonstrate Medicaid eligibility, the hospital may not have sufficient house physicians to provide the needed care.

3. *Inadequate accounting procedures.* If a hospital has inefficient bookkeeping and billing procedures, the hospital's capacity to take chances on admitting those with uncertain eligibility is reduced.[47]

A 10 year study of a cohort of welfare cases in New York City investigated the impact of Medicaid on access to medical care and utilization patterns. The old and very sick actually received less care under Medicaid than before its initiation. Under the previous welfare system, whatever its imperfections of quality or acceptability, recipients apparently had ready access to a doctor and made many visits. Fewer untreated conditions (both mild and severe) were found than after Medicaid was implemented. Medicaid seems to have benefited mostly the younger and less sick of the low income families studied. The proportion of persons from these groups seeing a doctor rose after the Medicaid program went into effect and the average number of physician visits increased.[48]

However, a study of Medicaid utilization among children in Rochester, New York, produced disturbing findings. Between 1967 and 1969 the number of Medicaid children with a private doctor *fell* from 45 to 30 percent. Children lacking a regular source of care rose from 22 percent to 39 percent. While middle-class children averaged 5.4 medical contacts per year, children on the Medicaid program had only 3.7 visits per year of which less than half were given by private practitioners. Medicaid enrolled children had 40 percent less preventive visits per year than Blue Cross registered children, and about 20 percent fewer illness related visits.[49] Part of the problem is a drop in Medicaid enrollment due to changed eligibility criteria in 1969 combined with discontinuance of the policy of reimbursing Medicaid providers at the level of usual and customary fees. Both accounted for a marked drop in the use of private physicians by Medicaid patients. However, even if the structure of the program had remained unchanged, it is clear that simply removing financial barriers to care will not eliminate socioeconomic differences in health care utilization. To really make the program a success, major efforts must be made to bring the consumers and providers of services together.

Health Services for American Indians

No discussion of health services for the poor would be complete without an examination of the comprehensive health care program operated by the Public Health Service on behalf of American Indians residing on reservations. With few exceptions reservation Indians are entitled to free medical care if they are of one-fourth or more Indian blood.

The nation's 450,000 reservation Indians form the most poverty stricken minority group in the United States. The median family income is less than $4,000 a year or less than a third of non-Indian median family income. Unemployment in 1972 was 40 percent of the reservation labor force or nearly eight times higher than the national average.[50]

Responsibility for the health care of Indians and Alaska natives was transferred on July 1, 1955, from the Bureau of Indian Affairs (BIA) to a special Division of Indian Health in the Public Health Service (PHS) of the U.S. Department of Health, Education and Welfare. It was thought that the Public Health Service would have greater success in recruiting physicians to work on reservations, partly because of higher salaries and better fringe benefits. Furthermore, Congress was not as hostile to HEW appropriations as to those of the BIA. Indian health has improved substantially in the nearly two decades since the transfer took place, largely because of increased appropriations, which have quintupled between 1955 and 1971.

A marked reduction in Indian infant mortality and deaths from infectious diseases has occurred since 1955. (See Table 7-6.) These statistics indicate the greater decline in infant, tuberculosis, and gastroenteritis death rates for Indians as compared with blacks and whites since that time. The Indian infant mortality rate has fallen significantly below that of blacks, implying greater access to health services by Indian mothers and infants, as well as more rapid improvement in housing and sanitation among the latter. In spite of the significant progress in reducing the infant death rate and the mortality rates from infectious diseases among reservation Indians, these death rates are still comparable to those among whites 15 to 20 years ago.

Table 7-6

Infant, Tuberculosis, and Gastroenteritis Death Rates: Reservation Indians, Whites, and Blacks, Selected Years, 1955-71

Year	Infant Death Rates (Per 1,000 Live Births)			Tuberculosis (Per 100,000 Population)			Gastroenteritis (Per 100,000 Population)		
	Indian	White	Black	Indian	White	Black	Indian	White	Black
1955	61	26.2	51.4	47	7.6	21.7	41	3.6	10.5
1957	57	25.9	50.9	34	6.7	17.3	35	3.7	10.3
1959	50	24.0	47.4	28	4.8	17.2	30	3.8	9.2
1961	44	22.5	40.8	25	3.8	14.0	28	3.7	8.4
1963	40	22.2	41.3	25	3.4	12.8	22	3.9	7.9
1965	37	20.9	40.2	19	2.8	10.9	20	3.7	6.7
1967	30	19.6	35.4	16	2.2	10.1	16	3.7	4.7
1969	26	18.4	31.6	12	1.6	7.2	15	3.9	4.5
1971	23	16.8	30.2	6	1.2[a]	5.0[a]	7	3.8[a]	4.4[a]
Percentage Change									
1955-71	−62	−35	−41	−87	−84	−77	−83	+0.6	−58

[a]Estimated.

Source: Indian statistics and infant mortality statistics from U.S. Public Health Service, *Indian Health Trends and Services*, 1974 edition (Washington, D.C.: U.S. Government Printing Office, 1974), pp. 22 and 24; other statistics for blacks and whites from U.S. Department of Health, Education, and Welfare, *Vital Statistics of the United States*, various annual volumes, 1963-1971.

While reductions in mortality rates among Indians from infectious diseases have been encouraging, the *incidence* of many infectious diseases has not declined notably. Although morbidity from tuberculosis, syphilis, and dysentery has fallen rapidly (more rapidly than for the non-Indian population), there have been large *increases* from 1952-54 to 1971 among reservation Indians in the incidence of hepatitis, pneumonia, influenza, and chickenpox.[51] Morbidity rates among Indians from most infectious diseases are far higher than for the non-Indian population. Thus, a reservation Indian is 9 times as likely as a non-Indian to contact tuberculosis; 54 times as likely to be stricken with dysentery; and 11 times as likely to contact hepatitis.

The principal causes of the high incidence of infectious disease among reservation Indians are their low socioeconomic status and substandard housing. According to a 1966 survey, 75 percent of all reservation homes are substandard with 50 percent so dilapidated as to be beyond repair.[52] On the Navajo reservation, where nearly one-fourth of the nation's reservation Indians live, only 20 percent of the homes have running water and adequate means of waste disposal and only 17 percent have electricity. Half of all the families use a potentially contaminated water source.[53]

To ameliorate some of the environmental health problems caused by poor housing and inadequate waste disposal, Congress passed the Indian Sanitation Facilities Act in 1959. As a result of this program some 78,000 reservation Indian families have been provided running water and indoor waste disposal systems. By 1972 half of all reservation homes had adequate sanitation facilities.[54] These facilities have been important in reducing the infant mortality rate and morbidity rate from selected infectious diseases. (See Table 7-6.)

Personnel

Increased appropriations by Congress resulted in an increase between 1955 and 1971 of more than 75 percent in total personnel in the Indian Health Division. Although the number of physicians and dentists increased 290 percent and 350 percent, respectively, there are still proportionately far fewer health personnel serving Indians than among the non-Indian population. (See Table 7-7.) In relative terms there are 50 percent more physicians for the general population as for reservation Indians, and more than two and one half times as many pharmacists. The lack of dentists and public health nurses is not as great: In 1970 there was one dentist for each 1,990 persons in the general population, compared with one for 2,520 reservation Indians; and one public health nurse for every 2,200 of the general population compared with one for every 2,800 reservation Indians.

Physicians applying for positions with the Division of Indian Health must have served a one-year internship in an accredited hospital. Nearly 70 percent of

Table 7-7
Number of Persons Served by Each Physician, Dentist, Public Health Nurse, and Pharmacist, 1955, 1962, and 1971

Profession	Indian Health Program			General Population
	1955	1962	1971	1971
Physician	2,200	1,460	990	660
Dentist	7,000	4,600	2,520	1,990
Public health nurse	4,000	3,500	2,800	2,200
Pharmacist	51,400	6,460	3,120	1,580

Sources: Data for 1955 and 1962 are from *A Review of the Indian Health Program*, Hearing before the Subcommittee on Indian Affairs of the House Committee on Interior and Insular Affairs, 88th Congress (1963), pp. 27 and 51; data for 1971 from U.S. Public Health Service *Indian Health Trends and Services*, 1974 Edition (Washington, D.C.: U.S. Goverment Printing Office, 1974), pp. 1 and 78; data for 1970, Public Health Service, *The Supply of Health Manpower, 1970 Profiles and Projections to 1990* (Washington, D.C.: U.S. Government Printing Office, 1974), p. 46.

the physicians and dentists in the Indian service have served there in lieu of military service, and few remain more than the required two years (the time draftees were required to serve in the armed services). There has been great turnover among staff, which affects program continuity. The principal reason has been the higher pecuniary rewards offered elsewhere although other factors such as isolation are important. A doctor or dentist entering the Indian Health Division in 1970 received a base salary of $13,400 a year, which could reach a maximum (with major administrative responsibility and twenty-six years service) of $24,000.[55] The average income in private practice in 1968 was $36,000 for physicians and an estimated $24,500 for dentists.[56]

Since most of the physicians employed by the Division of Indian Health are not specialists (nor is it likely that at the above pay scales many specialists could be attracted) patients requiring a specialist are usually referred to private physicians under contract in urban areas near the reservations. Funds for contract care have been adequate, so that the lack of specialists to provide health care for Indians is minimal.

Nurses who have graduated from a two-year college program are hired by the Indian Health Division at $7,000 a year. Those who have completed three or four-year programs entered at $7,400 in 1970. These salaries were reasonably competitive with non-Indian service alternatives in major metropolitan areas, where nurses generally received starting salaries ranging from $6,000 to $7,000 per year. However, to attract good nurses to some of the isolated locations requires higher salaries than they would receive elsewhere. A high rate of turnover among nurses will probably continue until more Indian RNs are brought into the service, since more of them would be familiar with this type of area and thus be less likely to object to such a location. At present, only a small percentage of Indian Health Service RNs are Indian, but the proportion has been rising in recent years.

Training Programs

It is the policy of the Division of Indian Health to train and employ as many Indians and Alaskan natives in its programs as possible. From 50 to 60 percent of the health personnel employed by the division are Indians, although the number of Indian physicians and dentists employed is less than 1 percent of all professional Indian personnel. Between 1955 and 1970 more than 1,500 Indians and Alaskan natives were trained for auxiliary positions, including practical nurses, dental and nursing assistants, sanitarian aides, community health aides, medical records technicians, and clerks. Moreover, on-the-job training is provided for service personnel, housekeepers, and ambulance drivers.

Health Facilities and Services

The Division of Indian Health operates 50 hospitals. Since 1955, 7 hospitals have been constructed and others have had extensive modernization. Seven obsolete ones have been closed. In spite of the improvement in facilities, only 20 of the 50 hospitals maintained by the Indian Health Division were accredited in 1968-69, because of lack of blood banks, inadequate separation of patients with various infectious diseases, and small size (hospitals with fewer than 25 beds were not eligible for accreditation).[57]

The Division of Indian Health also maintains health centers and stations—the centers are outpatient facilities staffed by full-time personnel and providing medical care and teaching preventive health measures. The stations that are intermittently staffed, hold scheduled clinics and supply medical care and other health services. Between 1955 and 1971, 17 centers and 58 stations were built.

Since 1955 there has been a rapid growth in the services provided under the program. Admissions to hospitals have increased more than 104 percent, and hospital outpatient visits have nearly quadrupled. By 1963, 97 percent of all Indian babies were born in hospitals, compared with 85 percent in 1952. Also, total outpatient visits to health centers and health stations increased nearly ninefold between 1951 and 1972. The level of dental services provided increased almost four times. The most rapid expansion took place in pharmaceutical services, which were virtually nonexistent when the Public Health Service took over the Indian health program.

Continuing Health Problems

One of the greatest needs is a well-developed mental health program. There is a high incidence of suicide on some reservations, especially among young people.[58] The need for trained psychiatrists and psychologists is critical.

In the past, only limited psychiatric services were available to Indians through contract arrangements made by the Division of Indian Health, and patients placed in state mental hospitals received only custodial care. In recent years, however, the division has begun to develop a mental health program. In 1965 a pilot project was established on the Pine Ridge Reservation in South Dakota. The staff included a psychiatrist, an anthropologist, a psychologist, and two aides.[59] In 1966 a psychiatrist, a psychologist, and a mental health social worker were added to the Anchorage area staff; this team provides services to all Indian hospitals and schools throughout the state. More recently, psychiatrists have been added to area offices at Phoenix, Albuquerque, and Window Rock. Compared with some of the other types of health services provided, however, the mental health program is still in its infancy.

Closely related to mental health is alcoholism, which is a serious health problem on the reservations and among urban Indians.[60] On some reservations and in western metropolitan areas over 90 percent of the arrests are alcohol related.[61] In 1971 the death rate from alcoholism among reservation Indians was 46.3 (per 100,000) compared with 7.5 (per 100,000) in the general population.[62] Most Indian hospitals have no special treatment facilities for alcoholism, which is generally treated as a crime, not an illness. Research into the causes of alcoholism among American Indians is badly needed. There appears to be a wide range of opinion concerning the high incidence of alcoholism, but little in the way of hard information.

A third problem is the lack of dental services to adults. Because of limited funding and personnel, most Indian service dentists devote the major part of their time to children. In 1973 less than 20 percent of the population aged 20 and over received dental treatment; about half of those under 20 were cared for.[63]

Summary

There is a strong negative relationship between mortality rates and income levels. Moreover, chronic illness resulting in activity limitation is also closely related to income level; the more severe the limitation, the stronger the association. However, research has also shown that poor health and more specifically disability, has resulted in low incomes and declines in socioeconomic status.

Neighborhood Health Centers have expanded rapidly in the past decade and presently serve about three million persons. They have generally succeeded in obtaining consumer involvement in their operations. In addition, the quality of care rendered compares favorably with that of other providers. However, many families are reluctant to make the centers their sole source of care. This is one factor that has limited the rise in the utilization level of health services by the poor.

The Medicaid program has grown rapidly since its inception and now is the second largest federal health program. However, a review of the literature indicates that the program's impact on utilization has been mixed. Eligibility restrictions and the refusal of some physicians to accept Medicaid patients have limited the effectiveness of the program.

Since 1955 health services for American Indians have been provided by the Public Health Service. While the health status of American Indians is becoming more similar to that of non-Indians, there is still a much greater incidence of infectious diseases among the former. Expansions in the mental health and dental care programs are badly needed as well as the development of an alcoholism treatment and prevention program.

Notes

1. Gordon F. Bloom and Herbert R. Northrup, *Economics of Labor Relations* (Homewood, Illinois: Richard D. Irwin, Inc., 1973), p. 448.

2. U.S. Department of Commerce, *Characteristics of the Low Income Population: 1971*, Consumer Income Series P-60, No. 82 (Washington, D.C.: U.S. Government Printing Office, 1972), p. 1.

3. Monroe Lerner, "Social Differences in Physical Health," in John Kosa, Aaron Antonovsky and Irving Zola (Eds.), *Poverty and Health A Sociological Analysis* (Cambridge, Massachusetts: Harvard University Press, 1969), p. 81.

4. Lerner, "Social Differences," p. 85.

5. Wayne E. Smith, "Factors Associated With Age–Specific Death Rates, California Counties, 1964," *American Journal of Public Health*, Vol. 58, October 1968, pp. 1937-49.

6. Harold Luft, *Poverty and Health: An Empirical Investigation of the Economic Interactions*, unpublished doctoral dissertation, 1972, p. 78.

7. Luft, *Poverty and Health*, p. 79. However, even where low income "causes" poor health, one must be aware of the importance of environmental and attitudinal variables.

8. William C. Richardson, "Poverty, Illness and Use of Health Services in the United States," *Hospitals*, Vol. 43, July 1, 1969, p. 35.

9. Ibid.

10. Elijah L. White, "A Graphic Presentation of Age and Income Differentials in Selected Aspects of Morbidity, Disability, and Utilization of Health Services," *Inquiry*, Vol. 5, March, 1968, p. 20.

11. Luft, *Poverty and Health*, p. 66.

12. White, "A Graphic Presentation," pp. 21-23.

13. U.S. Department of Health, Education and Welfare, National Center for Health Statistics, *Age Patterns in Medical Care, Illness and Disability, 1968-1969*, Series 10-70 (Washington, D.C.: U.S. Government Printing Office, 1972), p. 10.

14. U.S. Department of Health, Education and Welfare, National Center for Health Statistics, *Volume of Physician Visits, 1966-1967*, Series 10-49 (Washington, D.C.: U.S. Government Printing Office, 1968), p. 19.

15. Myron J. Lefcowitz, "Poverty and Health: A Re-Examination," *Inquiry*, Vol. X, No. 1, March 1973, p. 7.

16. Thomas Bice, Robert Eichhorn, and Peter Fox, "Socioeconomic Status and Use of Physicians' Services: A Reconsideration," *Medical Care*, May-June 1972, Vol. X, No. 3, p. 263.

17. Ronald Andersen and Lee Benham, "Factors Affecting the Relationship Between Family Income and Medical Care Consumption," in Herbert E. Klarman (Ed.), *Empirical Studies in Health Economics* (Baltimore, Maryland: The Johns Hopkins Press, 1970), p. 92.

18. W.C. Richardson, "Measuring the Urban Poor's Use of Physicians' Services in Response to Illness Episodes," *Medical Care*, Vol. 8, 1970, p. 138.

19. Thomas Bice, Medical Care for the Disadvantaged: A Survey of Use of Medical Services in the Baltimore SMSA, Baltimore, The Johns Hopkins University, 1971.

20. Paul O. Flaim, "Persons Not in the Labòr Force," Special Labor Force Report No. 110, U.S. Department of Labor, Bureau of Labor Statistics reprint from *Monthly Labor Review*, Vol. 92, July 1969, p. 11.

21. Herbert S. Parnes, et al., *The Pre-Retirement Years: A Longitudinal Study of the Labor Market Experience of Men*, Vol. I, Manpower Research Monograph No. 15 (Washington, D.C.: U.S. Government Printing Office, 1970), p. 99.

22. Luft, *Poverty and Health*, p. 189.

23. Ibid., p. 200.

24. Saad Z. Nagi and Linda Hadley, "Disability, Behavior: Income Change and Motivation to Work," *Industrial and Labor Relations Review*, Vol. 25, January 1972, p. 225.

25. P.S. Lawrence, "Chronic Illness and Socioeconomic Status," in E. Gartley Jaco (Ed.), *Patients, Physicians and Illness* (Glencoe, Illinois: Free Press, 1948), pp. 38 and 44.

26. Jerome L. Schwartz, "Early Histories of Selected Neighborhood Health Centers," *Inquiry*, Vol. 7, December 1970, p. 5.

27. Schwartz, "Early Histories," p. 4.

28. Economic Opportunity Act, as Amended; 42USC 2809. The specific authorization for the "Comprehensive Health Services Program" was originally included in 1966 as Section 211-2 and became Section 222(a)(4) through later amendments.

29. Daniel I. Zwick, "Some Accomplishments and Findings of Neighborhood Health Centers," *Milbank Memorial Fund Quarterly*, Vol. 50, October 1972, p. 390.

30. Gerald Sparer, George Dines, and Daniel Smith, "Consumer Participation in OEO-Assisted Neighborhood Health Centers," *American Journal of Public Health*, Vol. 60, June 1970, pp. 1091-1102.

31. Sparer, et al., "Consumer Participation," p. 1095.

32. Jerome L. Schwartz, *Medical Plans and Health Care: Consumer Participation in Policy Making* (Springfield, Illinois: Charles C. Thomas, 1968).

33. Geomet, Inc., *Study to Evaluate the OEO Neighborhood Health Center Program at Selected Centers* (Rockville, Maryland), Vol. 1, 1971, p. 12.

34. Gerald Sparer and Joyce Johnson, "Evaluation of OEO Neighborhood Health Centers," *American Journal of Public Health*, Vol. 61, No. 5, May 1971, pp. 935-36.

35. Mark Strauss and Gerald Sparer, "Basic Utilization Experience of OEO Comprehensive Health Services Projects," *Inquiry*, Vol. 8, December 1971, p. 44.

36. H.H. Tilson, "Stability of Physician Employment in Neighborhood Health Centers," *Medical Care*, Vol. 11, No. 5, September-October, 1973, p. 391.

37. Zwick, "Some Accomplishments," p. 407.

38. Sparer and Johnson, "Evaluation of OEO Neighborhood Health Centers," p. 940.

39. *Recommendations of the Task Force on Medicaid and Related Programs* (U.S. Department of Health, Education and Welfare, June 1970), processed, p. 16.

40. Robert J. Myers, *Medicare* (Homewood, Illinois: Richard D. Irwin, Inc., 1970), p. 268.

41. Karen Davis, "Lessons of Medicare and Medicaid for National Health Insurance," in *National Health Insurance—Implications*, Hearings before the Subcommittee on Public Health and Environment of the House Committee on Interstate and Foreign Commerce, 93rd Congress 1st and 2nd Session (1974), p. 214.

42. Bruce C. Stuart and Lee A. Bair, *Health Care and Income: The Distributional Impacts of Medicaid and Medicare Nationally and in the State of Michigan*, Research Paper No. 5 (State of Michigan: Department of Social Services, 1971), p. 42. Part of the difference is due to the larger sized families of the Medicaid recipient.

43. Barbara S. Cooper, Nancy L. Worthington, and Paula A. Piro, "National Health Expenditures, 1929-1973," *Social Security Bulletin*, Vol. 37, No. 2, February 1974, p. 8.

44. Ibid., p. 9.

45. Margaret C. Olendzki, Richard P. Grann, and Charles H. Goodrich, "The Impact of Medicaid on Private Care for the Urban Poor," *Medical Care*, Vol. 10, No. 3, May-June 1972, p. 204.

46. Dennis H. Leverett and Anthony Jong, "Variations in Use of Dental Care Facilities by Low Income White and Black Urban Populations," *Journal of the American Dental Association*, Vol. 80, No. 1, January 1970, p. 139.

47. Stephen M. Davidson and Ronald C. Wacker, "Community Hospitals and Medicaid," *Medical Care*, Vol. 12, No. 2, February 1974, pp. 126-27.

48. Margaret C. Olendzki, "Medicaid Benefits Mainly the Younger and Less Sick," *Medical Care*, Vol. 12, No. 2, February 1974, p. 163. The fact that utilization rates for the young improved is a positive finding, since utilization data indicate that physician visits are a positive function of family income for the young.

49. Klaus J. Roghmann, Robert Haggerty, and Rodney Lorenz, "Anticipated and Actual Effects of Medicaid on the Medical-Care Pattern of Children," *New England Journal of Medicine*, Vol. 285, No. 19, p. 1055.

50. Alan Sorkin, "Business and Industrial Development on American Indian Reservations," *Annals of Regional Science*, Vol. 7, No. 2, December 1973, p. 115.

51. U.S. Department of Health, Education and Welfare, *Indian Health Trends and Services*, 1974 Edition (Washington, D.C.: U.S. Government Printing Office, 1974), pp. 51-52. Part of the increase in the incidence of some diseases is due to improved case detection.

52. Task Force on Indian Housing, "Indian Housing: Need, Alternatives, Priorities and Program Recommendations," Bureau of Indian Affairs, December 1966, processed.

53. *Federal Facilities for Indians: Tribal Relations with the Federal Government*, Report by Mamie L. Mizen, Staff Member, Senate Committee on Appropriations, 1966, p. 455.

54. U.S. Department of Health, Education and Welfare, *Indian Health Trends and Services*, p. 1.

55. Unpublished tabulation, U.S. Public Health Service (salaries effective January 1, 1970).

56. Arthur Owens, "The New Surge in Physicians' Earnings and Expenses," *Medical Economics*, Vol. 46, December 8, 1969, p. 62.

57. Alan Sorkin, *American Indians and Federal Aid* (Washington, D.C.: The Brookings Institution, 1971), p. 62.

58. The age adjusted suicide rate among reservation Indians is at least 50 percent greater than among non-Indians. See Michael Ogden, Mozart Spector, and Charles Hill, Jr., "Suicides and Homicides Among Indians," *Public Health Reports*, Vol. 85, January 1970, p. 75.

59. Calvin A. Kent and Jerry W. Johnson, *Indian Poverty in South Dakota* (University of South Dakota, 1969), p. 111.

60. Maurice L. Sievers, "Cigarette and Alcohol Use by Southwestern American Indians," *American Journal of Public Health and the Nation's Health*, Vol. 58, January 1968, pp. 71-81.

61. For example, police records in Denver indicated that about half of the Negro migrants are arrested at least once during their stay in the city with about 95 percent of the arrests alcohol related. See T. Graves and M. Van Arsdale, "Values, Expectation and Relocation: The Navajo Migrant to Denver," *Human Organization*, Vol. 26, Winter, 1966, pp. 300-307.

62. U.S. Department of Health, Education and Welfare, *Indian Health Trends and Services*, p. 43.

63. U.S. Public Health Service, *Dental Services for American Indians and Alaska Natives, 1973* (Washington, D.C.: U.S. Government Printing Office, 1973), p. 16.

8 Health Insurance

Health insurance is a financial mechanism for spreading the costs of medical care over as large a proportion of the group at risk as possible. It is one method for removing all, or part, of the economic barrier to health and medical care services. The justification for health insurance is the uneven and unpredictable incidence of illness that leads to wide fluctuations in medical care expenditures at a point in time. One purpose of health insurance is to equalize the distribution of the burden of medical care costs among individuals and families. Because health insurance entails a transfer of purchasing power from the well to the sick, it increases the total demand for services. It also assures that the producer will be paid for services rendered.[1]

Health insurance began to show substantial growth toward the end of the nineteenth century with the entry of accident insurance companies into the field. Moreover, accident and health insurance also began to become available through life insurance firms.

At this time, the emphasis of health insurance was directed toward replacement of income rather than provision of hospital or surgical benefits. The early insurance company policy protected the policyholder against loss of earned income due to a limited number of diseases, including typhus, typhoid, scarlet fever, smallpox, diptheria, diabetes, and a few others. These policies contained a provision for a seven-day waiting period before the start of benefit payments. The benefit period was limited to 26 consecutive weeks.[2]

In 1929 a group of school teachers made an arrangement with Baylor Hospital in Dallas, Texas, to provide them with hospital care on a prepayment basis. This was the origin of the Blue Cross concept for the provision of hospital care, and it had a major effect on the health insurance industry by foreshadowing the development of the reimbursement policy for hospital and surgical care.

By 1938, 1.4 million people in the United States had enrolled in 38 Blue Cross health insurance plans. Private companies provided hospital insurance to only 100,000 people.[3] During the 1940s Blue Cross expanded rapidly, while the private health insurance industry also grew, but more slowly. Several factors contributed to the rapid growth of Blue Cross: It began writing contracts with employers having nationwide coverage; health insurance increasingly became a matter for collective bargaining, with labor supporting Blue Cross; and employment and wages increased rapidly during World War II. In 1945 Blue Cross claimed 61 percent of the hospital insurance market, compared with the insurance companies' 33 percent.

In the postwar period three factors interacted to spur the growth of the health insurance industry. First, the United States Supreme Court held that fringe benefits—including health insurance—were a legitimate part of the bargaining process in labor-management negotiations. Second, health care costs sharply escalated, which prompted the public to find a way to protect itself against the expense. The third force was the continuing improvement of health insurance itself through the introduction of new plans such as major medical insurance and the broadening of existing policies. For example, in recognition of changing social values, some group plans now include coverage for abortions, births out-of-wedlock, and vasectomies. Alcoholism and drug addiction are being covered with some policies including payment for treatment in a sanitarium. Psychiatric care, too, is available as a benefit in most group plans.

Two major characteristics have distinguished Blue Cross from most commercial insurance companies: payment of service benefits to hospitals rather than cash benefits to the person insured; and community rating, that is, the provision of benefits to all members of the community at the same rate, rather than higher rates to high risk groups. Since low-income families and the aged tend to utilize hospital services more than the general population, these groups are helped by community rating. As indicated above, during World War II, organized labor insisted on more adequate health benefits and other insurance companies began to compete for this growing business. Blue Cross substituted experience rating for community rating.[4] Today most Blue Cross plans offer group experience-rated contracts, particularly for larger group policies, as well as community-rated policies for those individuals who are not able to obtain a group policy at their place of employment.

The adoption of experience rating was probably inevitable if Blue Cross was to compete successfully with the commercial insurers for the business of the low-risk customer. There were two other possible options. The first would be to persuade low-risk groups that Blue Cross was so useful as an organization serving the entire community that low-risk customers should subsidize the costs of the higher risk groups. The second alternative would be to offer a service so excellent that high-risk groups could be subsidized without severe competitive disadvantage. Both of these possibilities would have been very difficult.

In 1972 private insurance met some of the cost of in-hospital physicians' visits and out-of-hospital x-ray and laboratory examinations for 72 percent of Americans, but far smaller numbers were reimbursed for other medical expenses. (See Table 8-1.) For example, only 53 to 56 percent of the civilian population was covered in any part for prescribed drugs, private-duty nursing, and visiting-nurse service. Moreover, only 22 percent had any insurance for nursing-home care; and less than 9 percent had any insurance to cover dental care. Insurance coverage for physicians' office and home visits, dental care, and drugs is subject to deductible and coinsurance payments; consequently, the full cost of these health care services is almost never met through insurance.

Table 8-1

Estimates of Net Numbers of Different Persons Under Private Health Insurance Plans and Percent of Population Covered, by Age and Specified Type of Care, as of December 31, 1972

Type of Service	All Ages		Under Age 65		Aged 65 and Over	
	Number (in Thousands)	Percent of Civilian Population	Number (in Thousands)	Percent of Civilian Population	Number (in Thousands)	Percent of Civilian Population
Hospital care	159,526	77.0	148,285	79.7	11,270	53.2
Physicians services:						
surgical services	153,326	74.0	143,525	77.1	9,813	46.3
in-hospital visits	149,734	72.2	141,579	76.1	8,155	38.5
x-ray and laboratory examinations	149,444	72.1	141,694	76.1	7,750	36.6
office and home visits	99,914	48.2	95,568	51.3	4,436	20.5
Dental care	17,904	8.6	17,608	9.5	296	1.4
Prescribed drugs (out of hospital)	111,374	53.7	107,855	58.0	3,519	16.6
Private duty nursing	108,959	52.6	105,518	56.7	3,441	16.3
Visiting nurse service	115,904	55.9	111,416	59.9	4,488	21.2
Nursing home care	45,460	21.9	39,987	21.5	5,473	25.8
HIAA estimates						
Hospital care	181,602	87.6	169,555	9.1	12,047	56.9
Surgical services	166,261	80.2	156,646	84.2	9,615	45.4

Source: Marjorie S. Mueller, "Private Health Insurance in 1972: Health Care Services, Enrollment and Finances," *Social Security Bulletin*, Vol. 37, No. 2, February 1974, p. 21.

In spite of the growth of private health insurance, in 1972 38 million Americans under age 65 still had no economic protection against hospital costs, and 43 million had no insurance for medical care costs. Although health insurance met 42 percent of all health care expenses in 1972, it paid for only 7 percent of consumer expenditures for health services other than those for hospital care and physician services. (See Table 8-1.)

In 1972 the private health insurance industry collected $22.3 billion in premiums and subscription charges from their policyholders and subscribers. A little more than 87 percent of the total was returned in claims and benefits.[5] Operating expenses amounted to $3.1 billion or 14 percent of premium income. The net underwriting loss was a little more than 1 percent of premium income, a loss made up for the most part in income from investments.

During 1972, insurance companies received almost $11 billion in premium income and Blue Cross-Blue Shield plans about $10 billion. However, the operating expenses of insurance companies were more than three times that of Blue Cross-Blue Shield plans—$2.3 billion or 21.4 percent of premium income, compared with 6.9 percent for Blue Cross-Blue Shield plans. The relatively high rate for insurance companies reflected mainly the operating expense ratio of 47 percent of premium income on individual policies.[6]

Insurance companies have relatively high acquisition costs and selling expenses and must pay federal and state taxes not required of the Blue Cross-Blue Shield plans. Moreover, insurance companies also write more than twice as much major medical insurance as do the Blue Cross-Blue Shield plans. The operating expense ratio on surgical-medical coverage is higher than the ratio on hospital coverage because of the lower premiums, the larger number of claims per enrollee, the smaller amount per claim, and the greater complexity of administering and paying surgical-medical claims in comparison with hospital claims. Major medical insurance is regarded as the most costly type of coverage to administer.

Insurance company group business and self-insured employer-employee union plans had the highest claim ratios; they returned 93 percent of premium income and 94 percent of subscription income, respectively in benefits. The rate of return on Blue Cross plans was close to that—92 percent. Individual insurance company policies paid only 53 cents in benefits for every premium dollar.[7]

As observed earlier, a fifth of the population under age 65 has no financial protection against illness. Still larger numbers have inadequate protection. Major deterrents are the cost and accessibility of health care services. Attempts to alleviate these problems are seen in the growing national interest in a system of universal health insurance and in the current emphasis of the federal government and health insurance industry on the new health maintenance organizations.

Health Maintenance Organizations

The term "Health Maintenance Organization" (HMO) refers to the following:

Generally an HMO is any organization that provides and assures the delivery of comprehensive health maintenance and treatment services for an enrolled group of persons under a prepaid, fixed capitation arrangement. Although the prepaid group practice concept is not new, what is new is the shift in emphasis in the HMO approach from acute episodic care to major concern for prevention of illness and maintenance of health. . . . The HMO's are designed to emphasize preventive medicine by providing incentives for cost consciousness and for increasing the productivity of available resources. They offer an opportunity for improving the quality of care. The HMO concept also offers a means for improving the geographic distribution of health services. By utilizing private capital and managerial talent, it is hoped that federal funding and direct controls can be reduced.[8]

Many health professionals would probably agree that two key deficiencies in the present health system are the organization of care and the type of incentives provided. The Health Maintenance Organization attempts to deal with these deficiencies. A good HMO program offers integrated, comprehensive care on both an ambulatory and inpatient basis. Competition is promoted between the physician and the traditional solo practitioner assuming relatively widespread HMO coverage.

Thus, an HMO, in addition to accepting payment for health care, assumes responsibility for actually providing health care services to its members. This is the major difference between an HMO and traditional health insurance. Health insurance pays part of the cost of health care while an HMO provides the services itself. Since it controls the delivery mechanism, an HMO, unlike indemnity insurance, is in a position to guarantee the availability, accessibility, and continuity of care.[9]

If the actual utilization of services is higher than predicted and costs are therefore above expected levels, the HMO must absorb the losses. Conversely, if utilization is below predicted levels, a surplus would result that either may be taken as profit or may be used to expand services to enrollees, and improve the quality of care. Unless there is some arrangement with an insurance company to assist with underwriting losses, an HMO must have a sufficiently large membership to allow dispersal of economic risk in order to avoid bankruptcy in the event of an epidemic or some catastrophic illness or disaster. The base enrollment necessary to obviate third party emergency underwriting is roughly 30,000 enrollees although the number can vary because of location and the characteristics of the enrollees.[10]

There are a number of advantages to the physician who is employed by an HMO. First, by participating in a group practice, he receives various types of fringe benefits such as low malpractice insurance rates, group life insurance, and sickness and retirement benefits. He has regular working hours. The physician is not concerned with the administrative details of operating his own business. Patient referral is easier than in private practice. The physician may benefit from the internal utilization process and from performance review by his peers. Another very important professional advantage is that since the HMO has a defined population base, the physician receives feedback from his patients and therefore can see how effectively he is practicing medicine from the consumers' viewpoint.

Some early evaluation studies indicate the effect of HMOs on the utilization of health services. Malcolm Peterson, investigating the Columbia (Maryland) Plan, reported that physicians' office visits were occurring at a rate of about 8.0 per person per year, compared with 4.6 nationally; hospital days by contrast were at a rate of 335 per 1,000 population per year, compared with about 1,100 days per 1,000 per year nationally.[11] Although these figures were not adjusted for age and socioeconomic status, they are still significant. A study by Milton I. Roemer indicated similar results. He found that the HMO investigated gave almost double the relative emphasis on ambulatory, compared with hospital bed service, than was the case for Blue Cross subscribers or enrollees in private health insurance plans.[12]

Another study in California examined the effect of family income on ambulatory care utilization under two HMO patterns: both the prepaid group practice (the Ross-Loos Medical Clinic Plan) and the medical care foundation (San Joaquin County) patterns. The study found that in both these HMO patterns, the effect of income was virtually nil—eliminating the correlation sometimes found between poverty and low utilization of outpatient services.[13]

With regard to expenditures by consumers or costs to patients, Roemer produced data on a prepaid group practice HMO in California, and compared it with conventional patterns. He analyzed annual expenditures by family units for physician and hospital services in terms of (a) insurance premiums, and (b) out-of-pocket expenditures. The results were as follows:[14]

Plan-Type	Average Premium	Out-of Pocket Expenditure	Total Costs
Commercial	$208	$156	$364
Blue Cross	257	190	447
HMO	271	52	323

Thus, while the average family premium of the HMO-type plan is higher the out-of-pocket expenditures for medical and hospital services are so much lower than in the other two plan types that total costs are lowest for the HMO enrollees. When family size is held constant the same general findings prevail.[15]

The ultimate measure of HMO performance is how healthy these organizations keep their members compared with other patterns of medical care delivery. Robert L. Robertson studied work loss in 1966-67 among school teachers covered by an HMO, compared with teachers covered by Blue Cross. The overall age-standardized mean days of work loss were 3.88 days per year in the HMO-type plan for males compared with 4.01 days in the Blue Cross plan; the parallel figures for females were 5.93 days compared to 6.41 days.[16]

The Blue Cross-Blue Shield plans have been active in forming, creating and expanding HMOs. In some instances Blue Cross plans have received federal grants for studies to determine the feasibility of implementing the HMO concept and for establishing HMO programs. The Blue Cross-Blue Shield plans have also instituted pilot programs and group-practice experiments. They have contracted with existing clinics and medical centers to convert part of their fee-for-service programs into a prepaid group practice.

By the end of 1972 more than 30 insurance companies had some degree of active involvement or exploratory interest in 50 operational or developmental HMOs in 22 states.[17] Involvement ranged from planning, administration, and marketing to financial support and/or underwriting a portion of the prepaid program in communities of all sizes.[18] Generally, the pattern has been to offer the HMO (prepaid) coverage to policyholders as an option to indemnity coverage.

On December 31, 1972, there were nine federally funded operational HMOs. Sixty-seven active grants for the planning and development of specific HMO's had been made. In addition funding was given to 47 projects designed to provide technical assistance in evaluating program efforts, to study HMO resources nationally, and to identify key factors in HMO development. A total of $25.9 million in grants and contracts has been obligated by the federal government since June 1971. Of this total, $16.9 million was for the direct support of HMO projects.[19]

The new HMO law signed on December 29, 1973, by President Nixon, is intended to stimulate the development of 100 to 150 new Health Maintenance Organizations. It is a major piece of health legislation. It pre-empts most of the state laws that have previously discouraged the development of HMO-type plans.[a] It authorizes $325 million in grants, loans, and loan guarantees to assist the development of HMOs. Moreover, the law requires employers to offer them as an optional form of health coverage for employees. This provision, called "mandatory dual choice" will affect every employer of 25 or more persons subject to minimum wage laws.[20]

Prepaid Plans—Case Studies

1. *Labor Union Plans:* As indicated previously, during World War II, labor unions obtained health benefits in their collective bargaining agreements. However, union members still could not always afford adequate medical care. Three direct service plans are illustrative of union attempts to meet this problem.

The Labor Health Institute of St. Louis is a prepaid group practice that seeks to provide high quality comprehensive care with an emphasis on prevention for

[a]Some state laws forbid prepaid group practice and do not permit Medicaid beneficiaries to join health insurance plans of the HMO type.

the union member and his family. However, the best known of these union programs was developed by the United Mine Workers for miners living in poor communities with inadequate facilities and limited educational opportunities. Supported by the union welfare fund and by royalties based on the amount of coal mined, the organization eventually built a chain of 10 hospitals in Kentucky, West Virginia, and Virginia (all subsequently sold). Unlike the St. Louis plan, which hired its own doctors, the welfare fund first tried to work with existing hospitals and doctors in a given area. However, the discrepancies in hospital admissions, length of stay, bills, and surgical procedures, in comparison with nonminers and their families, were so great that many doctors were separated from the program.[21] Benefiting from the experience of these earlier programs, the United Auto Workers in Detroit established the Community Health Organization and salaried their own physicians. They organized a prepaid comprehensive plan committed to high quality care, group practice coordinated by one's doctor, purchase of Metropolitan Hospital, and formation of three clinic centers in outlying areas.

2. *The Kaiser Program:* The Kaiser Foundation Medical Care Program has become the largest group practice prepayment plan in America. It has a membership of 2.2 million people. Presently the Kaiser plan operates in six regions—California, Oregon, Washington, Hawaii, Cleveland, and Denver. The plan employs 2,000 physicians and 13,000 nonphysicians who work in 22 hospitals and 51 clinics.[22]

The basic principles of the Kaiser-Permanente Medical Care Program are the organization of health care services (group medical practice with integrated health care facilities), voluntary enrollment, prepayment for services, comprehensive benefits provided on a direct-service basis, and preventive medical care with emphasis on early detection of disease. Revenue from subscribers is turned over to the physicians and hospitals (not as a fee for specific services). Thus, the physician has the incentive to keep the subscriber well and out of the hospital. Another principle is freedom of choice. Voluntary enrollment, with periodic options to change plans, permits every subscriber to select the type of health benefit plan that is most satisfactory for him; he can transfer to another plan if he is dissatisfied. In fact, it is Kaiser's policy to participate only in groups that provide such choices for their employees. Finally, the physician must be involved in the administration and operational decisions that affect the quality of care provided.

The average member's medical costs are 20 to 30 percent less than if he had obtained health services outside of the Kaiser system. The general population averages 137.9 hospital admissions a year per 1,000 people, while Kaiser admissions average 80 per 1,000 population. The national average for patient stay is 7.8 days compared with Kaiser's average patient stay of 6.65 days.[23] Thus, Kaiser's cost control is due primarily to the elimination of unnecessary health care, particularly hospitalization, which is achieved by its emphasis on illness prevention and early disease detection.

One major weakness of this plan is the lack of psychiatric services. Other areas that are excluded are dental care and the treatment of alcoholism and drug abuse. Moreover, Kaiser physicians indicate that they have not yet been able to give the proper emphasis to preventive medicine. This is because they have found it difficult to keep up with the rising demand for curative health services. Finally, the Kaiser Plan has been unable to enroll a significant number of poor persons.

3. *The Health Insurance Plan of Greater New York:* Featuring a prepaid insurance system that covers physician services and some clinical procedures, the Health Insurance Plan (HIP) of New York is characterized by peer control of the quality of services. A 28 member board of directors issues through its director of professional standards for medical group centers a set of guidelines concerning the level of quality at which member physicians must perform. The physicians are accountable to each other, and member groups are compared for their performance.

HIP is simply an insuring mechanism providing subscribers with 30 or so independent medical groups that are remunerated on an annual capitation basis.[24] At present, in addition to the medical groups, HIP has 41 medical centers and 1,160 doctors to serve the 783,000 enrollees. Like the Kaiser program, the consumer's wishes are expressed through a diverse board of directors, whose members—for example, union representatives—may speak in behalf of those consumers like themselves. Aside from this, subscriber dissatisfaction is expressed solely by choosing an alternative health plan.[25] Densen compared the experience of families insured under HIP with that of families insured under Group Health Insurance, Inc. The latter contracts with physicians in their private offices, pays them on a fee-for-service basis, and permits enrollees free choice of any licensed physician in New York City. The study found that (1) GHI enrollees had a higher age-sex adjusted hospital admission rate (8.8 per 100) than for HIP enrollees (7.0 per 100). The former also stayed longer in the hospital; (2) GHI subscribers had higher utilization of surgical procedures—both in and out of hospital; (3) the physician visit rate (but excluding surgical and obstetric visits) in home, office, and hospital was about the same for both groups.[26]

John M. Glascow has written persuasively that one should be cautious in adopting the prepaid group practice arrangement as national policy. He points out that any group practice will be designed to serve the interests of those that control it. "Since many groups have been formed by physicians it should be clear that the primary purpose of these particular groups is to meet physicians' needs. As a result there is no reason to expect that any savings in the physician dominated or owned group will be passed on to the consumer. Second, the resulting organization may not conform to patient or society views on the proper delivery form."[27] Depending upon one's definition of acceptance, the reported data on choice of prepaid group coverage by potential subscribers having alternative choices also strongly suggests evidence of resistance. However, the wide range in the percentage of persons eligible for membership who actually join—from as low as 2 percent to as high as 80 percent, as reported in various studies—does not allow definitive conclusions. It is evident, however, that acceptance of prepaid groups depends significantly on the absence of a prior patient-physician relationship.[28]

National Health Insurance

National health insurance is fundamentally a nationally organized financial mechanism based on social risk sharing. It is a public system for the collective financing of privately provided services.

There are few, if any, unresolved issues of social reform that have a lengthier or more turbulent history than national health insurance. Commissions to study the feasibility of social health insurance were formed in several states as early as 1910 to 1915. At this time the American Medical Association favored National Health Insurance: "The failure of many persons in this country at present to receive medical care constitutes the best argument for a change to the more effectual provision of medical attention offered by health insurance."[29]

On a national level a plan for financing health care was first mentioned in the presidential campaign of 1912 when it was an important plank in the platform of the Progressive party headed by Theodore Roosevelt.

Because of the first World War, attention was turned away from social legislation. Moreover, the conservative mood of the nation during the 1920s limited discussion of national health insurance. Thus, it was not until 1932 that the issue was resurrected by the Committee on the Cost of Medical Care, which recommended substantial changes in the nation's health system.[30] However, the committee, while it recommended in its majority report financing through comprehensive group payment, placed its reliance on voluntary action and refrained from recommending compulsory public health insurance.[31] By this time the American Medical Association had become firmly opposed to health insurance. "To recommend that our own country again experiment with discredited methods of voluntary insurance is simply to ignore all that has been learned by costly experience in many other countries as well as our own."[32]

During the 1920s the stance of organized labor was also hostile to social insurance. It was not until 1932 that the AFL formally withdrew its opposition to social insurance, and then only on condition that the costs be borne entirely by the employer.

The next opportunity to seriously consider national health insurance came in 1934-35, but the Committee on Economic Security did not include any proposals for health insurance in the proposed Social Security legislation, because the administration felt that the inclusion of so controversial a plan might endanger the passage through Congress of the old-age and unemployment insurance provisions.

The active opposition of the medical profession combined with the shift of priorities away from health associated with the Depression and World War II led to another period of dormancy. However, in 1943 the Wagner-Murray-Dingell Bill proposing universal health insurance attracted widespread interest among health experts.

The national health insurance issue reached its peak of public comment and legislative controversy in 1949. That year President Truman called for compulsory health insurance in his State of the Union Message. To counter the president's influence, the American Medical Association (AMA) launched a $1 million opposition campaign financed by a special assessment on its members.[33]

Congress gave extensive consideration to the issue in a highly charged atmosphere, but in the end no health insurance bill was passed. However, Congress did amend the Social Security Act to provide federal matching grants to the states for "vendor payments," with funds going directly to doctors, nurses, and health care institutions for the treatment of persons receiving public assistance.

Although President Truman repeated his request in 1950, national compulsory health insurance soon disappeared as a significant legislative issue. It reemerged about 10 years later in the form of health insurance for the elderly.

Beginning in the late 1960s the movement for national health insurance has again gained momentum resulting in the introduction of 16 different bills dealing with this issue in the 93rd Congress.[34]

If the United States had not been experiencing severe medical price inflation, the national health insurance issue might never have reached its present degree of public and legislative interest. General public awareness of our cost dilemma perhaps was associated with the Medicare and Medicaid programs, which have grown explosively in terms of funding; however, rapid increases in medical care costs antedate the Medicare and Medicaid programs. (See Chapter 1.)

While health care costs have been mounting, so have the expectations of Americans regarding health care. For example, the poor are disillusioned by the lack of geographic and financial availability of care; they expect more than has been provided under federal-state Medicaid programs. Thus, in 1970, for those Americans earning less than $3,500 per year, Welfare, Medicare, and Medicaid programs paid only one-half of all medical expenses.[35]

Although cost problems have been the major force toward increasing public interest in national health insurance, another factor is dissatisfaction with the current system of health care delivery. In fact, it is likely that the *kind* of national health insurance to be enacted will be influenced most strongly by this latter consideration. The fragmented organization of health care delivery, including a variety of specialists with no apparent linkages with other health professionals, and the difficulties in obtaining primary care seem to be perceived by an increasing proportion of the populace as evidence of a system organized to benefit the provider and not the consumer.[36]

As mentioned previously, private insurance covers almost 90 percent of the civilian population under 65 years of age and pays for approximately two-fifths of the health expenditures of those covered. Although insurance companies and Blue Cross-Blue Shield plans offer more liberal benefits, group and individual purchasers have generally been unwilling to pay the higher premiums necessary to expand benefits. Thus, private coverage is presently unable to meet the country's health care financing needs. However, one must remember that even if national health insurance becomes a reality, it cannot resolve certain health care problems. Thus, the manpower shortage in some health professions and the maldistribution of health personnel are among the difficulties that will have to be resolved independently of the health care financing system.

Criteria for Evaluating National Health Insurance Proposals

As indicated above, a large number of national health insurance proposals were introduced in the past session of Congress. How can they be compared and evaluated? Robert D. Eilers has indicated six major criteria that a national health insurance program should include.[37]

1. *Financial accessibility.* A national health insurance proposal should insure adequate medical care for all Americans regardless of economic status. The standard implies that those who are poor will incur virtually no personal expenses for most medical services.

The term "adequate care" should be interpreted narrowly at first, and broadened over time in order that increased demand does not overwhelm the supply of services available. However, a substantial portion of health care expenses should be paid immediately upon implementation. This would imply, according to Eilers, benefits covering roughly 50 percent of medical expenditures initially, increasing the next 10 years to a level of 80 percent of average total expenditures.[38]

2. *Delivery acceptability.* The system for delivering health services must meet with consumer approval and comprehension. The function of a national health insurance program goes beyond simply the pooling of total program costs over a wide population base. That is, the program should encourage the establishment of a health delivery system that results in greater utilization of all health services by some population segments (e.g., the poor), increased use of some services (e.g., preventive) by all population groups, and less use of some services (e.g., inpatient hospital care) by most segments of the population.

3. *Cost efficiency.* A national health insurance program must directly encourage consumer use of delivery arrangements that will make the most efficient use of the financial and human resources available. Although it may be difficult for some medical professionals to accept the change, it seems clear that national health insurance will cause an alteration in the methods of payment for health

services. "Specifically, a program must assure a phased movement toward at least partial capitation payment for services. Moreover, the capitation approach must not be applied separately to physicians' services and hospital services, but, rather, a single capitation to the responsible organization."[39]

The cost efficiency criterion requires that the impact of a national insurance program must extend beyond merely influencing the use of services through the benefits provided. Thus, national health insurance must exert a more direct influence on the nature of the delivery system.

4. *Minimization of government regulation.* A universal health insurance program should stimulate accountability and self-regulation by the financing and delivery system and should minimize the need for extensive government regulation. This goal can be achieved if consumers have the choice of obtaining the services, through one of several delivery organizations. Competition among these organizations will provide an incentive for organizational accountability of covered services. Consumer choice of delivery organization, coupled with capitation payment, will help achieve a self-regulating delivery system.

5. *Consumer participation in cost.* The majority of persons covered by national health insurance should pay a part of the cost of health services. This will minimize excessive use as well as the administrative costs associated with the program. Consumer participation in the basic financing, whether through a premium or taxation approach, will add to the funds available for health care, since employers cannot pay the entire cost for those in the labor force and their dependents without creating strong inflationary pressures. Employers will resist major increases in expenditures above the premiums (for private insurance) and taxes (for Medicare) that they are now paying, and employer lobbies may be able to cause Congress to turn down a national health insurance proposal if the employer is expected to pay the entire cost. However, general tax revenues should not be the sole or primary source of financing for national health insurance, since this would subject the program unnecessarily to the vicissitudes of legislative pressures. For example, in years when other needs were considered by Congress to be of major importance, the health program could be constricted if federal funds were the primary financial support.

Consumer cost participation has more advantages with less negative results if coinsurance is used in place of a deductible. If the nonpoor consumer bears a certain proportion, such as 15 or 20 percent of the direct cost of the service, he has substantial incentives for not making unnecessary use of health services.[40] Furthermore, the administrative costs are appreciably less than those associated with the deductible.

6. *Quality of care.* The national health insurance program should impose requirements of high quality care. The program should specify an increasingly rigorous surveillance of quality, with the basic guidelines of quality control being established by the federal government. Consumer desires concerning such items as waiting periods for physician office visits, and availability of nighttime care,

should be incorporated into the quality standards. However, any reviews of diagnoses or methods of treatment should continue to be made by health professionals.

National Health Insurance Proposals

Current proposals for national health insurance include provisions pertaining to eligibility, benefits, allowable delivery arrangements, and regulation. (The features of seven current proposals are summarized in Table 8-2.) Each of the proposals is discussed in terms of the six criteria discussed above.

In two of the current proposals (C and F), a tax incentive is used to stimulate the voluntary purchase of private health insurance. These would give employers or consumers who purchase "acceptable" private health insurance either a credit against their federal income tax or a deduction from their income subject to federal tax; acceptable insurance includes specified minimum benefits.

In proposal F, known as the Medicredit Plan, which is supported by the American Medical Association, the credit against the income tax would be a portion of the premium paid, such credit varying with the individual or family personal tax level. Families with a federal tax liability of $1,300 or more would be allowed a credit of only 10 percent of the premium, whereas those with a tax of $300 or less would have a credit for the entire premium.

Incentive-type proposals for national health insurance would give persons below the poverty level a federal certificate for national health insurance to obtain coverage from a private insurer of their own choice at no cost to themselves. The tax incentive proposals probably would have little effect on current financing and delivery arrangements. Moreover, there would be little government involvement in the programs. Tax-type proposals meet two criteria: minimization of government regulation and participation of the consumer in cost. However, since the cost of health care is a substantial motivation for national health insurance, it seems likely that tax credit plans in the long run would tend to stimulate increased government regulation because of the inability of these plans to deal with rising health care costs.

Tax incentive plans do not meet the criteria of delivery acceptability and cost efficiency. Thus, national health insurance based solely on a plan to stimulate the purchase of private insurance would provide no incentive to improve the health care delivery system through increased efficiency and greater consumer acceptance. Tax credit proposals meet part of the criterion of financial accessibility, assuming that minimum benefits require substantial coverage.

Certain proposals such as A and B make mandatory the purchase of private insurance on behalf of specified categories of persons. The compulsory private coverage proposals will help somewhat to increase accessibility and tend to meet the criteria of consumer participation in cost. Moreover, alternatives to the present health care delivery system are likely since employers who must finance the proposal will want to minimize their own costs. Small business would be most affected by a compulsory-private approach since they would be required to make the largest increases in their benefits to comply with the legislation. Since phased implementation is necessary under either the tax incentive or compulsory approach, it appears that minimum benefits would have to be lower under the compulsory coverage approach than the tax incentive approach (optional coverage). That is the delivery system would not have the capacity to deliver services if high minimum benefits were mandated under a compulsory-coverage arrangement.[41]

The administration estimates that the benefit package designed in the plan (proposal A) would require a total premium of approximately $600 for a family and $240 for an individual. Recognizing that the $450 contributed to the premium might significantly increase payroll expenses, the plan provides for a federal subsidy (declining over a five-year period) to employers for a portion of the premium costs in excess of 3 percent of total cash wages. Even with the maximum subsidy, an employer whose employees elected coverage for themselves and their families and who had average annual wages of $7,500 would find the wage bill increased 3.5 percent the first year and 6 percent by the fifth year. It is likely that these costs would be borne by the employee in reduced wages as are other payroll taxes.[42] Moreover, the program has other regressive characteristics: a premium that is a fixed dollar amount comprises a higher percentage of low incomes than of high incomes. Thus, married employees with an annual income of $7,500 would pay a 2 percent "tax" to meet their share of premium costs; for those with incomes of $75,000 the tax would be 0.2 percent.[43] Although few persons would reach the maximum—an individual would have to receive at least $3,600 worth of covered medical services before reaching the $1,500 liability limit (see Table 8-2)—the presence of such a maximum would offer a measure of security. However, by not relating benefits or premiums to income creates an impossible situation. A working family with an income of $7,500 would have a maximum liability of 20 percent of income, while one with $15,000 would have a 10 percent limit, and one with an income of $75,000 would have a 2 percent ceiling.[44] Moreover, the limits are not adjusted to take account of family size or the net worth of an individual.

The subsidy proposals have another shortcoming. The maximum amount of the insurance subsidy under the various plans is below the average premiums required for a fully comprehensive health insurance policy. Since the subsidy plans are generally intended to replace Medicaid and Medicare, which in some states provide relatively comprehensive coverage, subsidized private insurance would leave some low-income people worse off.[45]

Catastrophic coverage (proposal G) has similarities to major medical policies now sold by private insurance agencies. While proposal G contemplates using federal revenues for financing, other plans have suggested financing by payroll tax.

Table 8-2
Features of National Health Insurance Proposals

A. Comprehensive Health Insurance Act of 1974	B. National Health Care Services Reorganization and Financing Act	C. National Health Care Act of 1973
(Administration Proposal)		
Summary: Three-part program including (1) a plan requiring employers to provide private health insurance for employees, (2) an assisted plan for low-income and high-medical-risk populations, (3) improved Medicare for the aged program.	Three-part program including (1) plan requiring employers to provide private coverage for employees, (2) plan for individuals, (3) federal contracted coverage for poor and aged.	Three-part *voluntary* insurance plan: (1) an employee-employer plan, (2) a plan for individuals, (3) a state plan for the poor.
Benefits: No limit on hospital inpatient and outpatient services or physicians services. Deductibles of $150 per person and 25% coinsurance but total cost sharing limited to $1,500. However, cost sharing reduced for low-income persons.	Benefits phased in over five-year period. Hospitals 90 days, $5 payment per day; 90 days in nursing home ($2.50 copayment per day); 10 physician visits per year; $2 copayment per visit; catastrophic coverage available when certain noncovered expenses reach a certain level, which varies by family income and age.	Minimum benefits phased in over six-year period eventually to include 300 days in hospital ($10 deductible first day and $5 thereafter); 180 days in nursing home ($2.50 deductible per day); surgery unlimited physicians outpatient ($2 deductible per visit) no deductibles or copayment for poor.
Administration: Insurance through private carriers; assisted plan administered by states through private carriers; plan for aged administered in same way as Medicare.	Private insurance carriers under state supervision, according to federal guidelines; for low-income persons government contracts with private insurance carriers.	Insurance administered by private carriers under state supervision.
Financing: Employer-employee premium payments with employer paying 75% of premiums; premium payments for poor based on family income (none for lowest income groups); continuation of present Medicare financing for aged persons. Federal revenues used to finance cost sharing and premiums for low-income aged.	Employer-employee premium payments with employer paying 75%. Federal subsidy for payments by low-income workers and medically indigent. Balance of cost financed by federal general revenues and the payroll taxes of present Medicare program.	For employer-employee plan premium paid by employers and employees. Employees and employers and individuals can deduct entire premium from income tax; federal and state governments pay balance of costs from general revenues.

Delivery: Prepaid practice plans. Under all plans, option available to enroll in approved prepaid group.

Provider Payment: Reasonable charges to providers subject to Medicare limitations. Group practice systems on incentive capitation basis. Relies on market competition.

D. National Health Insurance and Health Services Improvement Act of 1973

Summary: Program based on expansion of Medicare to entire population. Also includes option for alternative coverage under private insurance plans.

Benefits: Same as Medicare, plus additional benefits. Most services (except institutional) subject to present Medicare "Part B" cost sharing of $60 annual deductible per person and 20% coinsurance.

Administration: Similar to Medicare, DHEW would have general administrative responsibility. Private insurance carriers (or quasi governmental corporations) would handle claims and pay providers.

Financing: Tax on payroll plus income from federal general revenues; tax rates: (a) 3.3% of earnings for employers, employees, and the self-employed, (b) general revenue contribution equal to one-half of total tax receipts.

Health care corporations that furnish all covered services, through its facilities or affiliated providers.

For health care corporations, a state commission would prospectively approve charges; for physicians and other professionals, reimbursement is based on reasonable fees, or salaries as approved by state commission.

E. Health Security Act (Kennedy-Griffiths Proposal)

A program providing broad benefits administered by federal government and financed by payroll taxes and federal general revenues.

Benefits with virtually no limitations; skilled nursing facility, 120 days of care.

Federal government. Special board in DHEW, with regional and local offices to operate program.

Tax on payroll, self-employed, and unearned income, and federal general revenues. (a) Tax rates 1% on employee wages and unearned income, (b) 3.5% for employers, (c) 2.5% for self-employed, and (d) federal general revenues equal to receipt from taxes.

Health maintenance organizations; must be made available as an option to persons enrolled in state plan and employer or employee plans.

Hospitals prepare budgets and charges reviewed by state commission and HEW, physicians and dentists are reimbursed on the basis of reasonable charges.

F. Health Care Insurance Act of 1973

Would provide credits against personal income taxes to offset the premium cost of health insurance. Employers are required to provide health insurance to retain favorable tax treatment.

Tax credits of 10 to 100% of cost of qualified health insurance; hospital care, $50 deductible per stay; physicians services, 20% coinsurance.

Private insurance carriers issue policies. State insurance departments certify carriers and qualified policies. A new federal board establishes standards for the program.

Tax credits financed by federal government. Employers must provide qualified policies as a condition of taking the full premium cost as a normal business deduction.

186

Table 8-2 (cont.)

D. National Health Insurance and Health Services Improvement Act of 1973 (cont.)	E. Health Security Act (Kennedy-Griffits Proposal) (cont.)	F. Health Care Insurance Act of 1973 (cont.)
Delivery: Comprehensive health service systems. DHEW can contract with comprehensive systems to provide health care to enrolled population. Systems must provide all covered services, preventive services, health education, and must train paramedical health personnel.	Health resources development fund will ultimately receive 5% of total income of program to be used to improve delivery; health maintenance organizations.	No provisions.
Provider Payment: Same as Medicare; new payment methods may be established after 1-2 years, based on a study required by bill.	Hospitals on the basis of approved prospective budgets. Group practice systems by complex incentive-based capitation. Fee for services strongly discouraged.	Usual and customary charges to all providers. No premium cost limits on carriers. Reliance on market competition.

G. National Catastrophic Illness Act of 1973

Summary: Program would pay medical expenses when they exceed a specified amount.

Benefits: All services eligible as medical expense deductions under the income tax law may be covered after family medical expenses exceed a specified amount.

Administration: Private insurance carriers would issue and administer the insurance policies. DHEW would establish regulations for the program.

Financing: Policyholders would pay premium. Premium rate: DHEW would determine actuarial value of policies, but could set a premium rate lower than the actuarial value to encourage widespread enrollment. It would pay carriers (from general revenues the difference between the actuarial value and the premium rate).

Delivery: No provisions.

Provider Payment: No provisions.

Source: Saul Waldman, *National Health Insurance: Provisions of Bills Introduced in the 93rd Congress as of February 1974*, U.S. Department of Health, Education, and Welfare, Publication No. 11920 (Washington, D.C.: U.S. Government Printing Office, 1974), pp. 4-16.

One important difficulty with the catastrophic approach is that such plans always impose fairly large deductibles and thus fail to meet the criterion of financial accessibility. This is because there is no assurance that even middle-income persons will believe they can afford such coverage.

Moreover, this proposal also fails to meet the cost efficiency criterion. It is assumed that medical services would be utilized efficiently because consumers have out-of-pocket expenses, and hence that patients would not overutilize health services. This contention may be incorrect. This type of policy relates solely to the financing of health care and thus does not stimulate greater efficiency in the delivery system.

The Javits Bill (proposal D) to extend Medicare to cover the entire population would be financed equally by employees, employers, and the federal government. Employees and employers would contribute on a tax base of $15,000 with a contribution by each reaching a level of 3.3 percent by 1975.

An extension of Medicare would meet the financial accessibility criteria, since the Medicare benefits are already extensive. In addition, consumers would participate in the cost of the plan both through the tax on wages and through the deductible and coinsurance provisions. The basic financing would not be a burden on the poor, even though the tax tends to be regressive because the tax rates would be low and apply only to those having earned income. The approximately equal sharing of the cost among workers, employers, and the federal government is not unreasonable since it shifts one-third of the cost to federal funds, which are obtained from a progressive tax structure.

However, it is unlikely that an expansion of Medicare would result in a delivery system that is more acceptable to consumers than present arrangements, nor would cost efficiency necessarily result. In addition, this proposal would require an extension of the detailed type of government regulation of the medical care industry now evolving under Medicare.

The Health Security Act (proposal E) anticipates coverage of virtually all citizens under an arrangement where the government would be intimately involved in the organization and administration of the delivery system. This proposal includes employer, employee, and governmental financing—with the employee paying the smallest share. (See Table 8-2.) This bill would result in the elimination of private insurers, at least in terms of present operations. The broad benefits proposed, and the possible extensive changes in the health delivery system would have to be phased in or else resources would be inadequate to meet demand. In addition, this legislation would establish an elaborate network of government regulation rather than a self-regulating health system. As one might expect, this proposal has provoked the greatest opposition among the medical profession of all the proposals considered, primarily because it discourages payment on a fee-for-service basis and because of the extensive government regulation required.

Table 8-3 summarizes the discussion of the various types of health insurance proposals in terms of the criteria developed by Eilers and discussed above.

Table 8-3

Evaluation of National Health Insurance in Relation to Suggested Criteria

Criterion	Tax Incentive Proposals	Compulsory Coverage Through Private Insurers	Catastrophic Coverage	Extension of Medicare	Compulsory Coverage Under Federally Administered System
Financial accessibility	–?	+(if nationwide adoption)	—	+	+
Delivery acceptability	—	+?	—	–?	+?
Cost efficiency	—	?	—	–?	?
Phased implementation	+	?	NA	+?	–
Consumer participation in cost	+	+	+	+	+?
Minimization of governmental regulation	–?	?	–?	–?	–
Quality of care	—	?	—	–?	+

Source: Robert D. Eilers, "National Health Insurance: What Kind and How Much," (Part II), *New England Journal of Medicine*, Vol. 284, No. 17, April 29, 1971, p. 953. Reprinted by permission of the *New England Journal of Medicine*.

Financial accessibility and consumer participation in cost appear to be the criteria most easily satisfied by the above proposals. The most difficult criteria to meet are delivery acceptability, cost efficiency, and minimization of governmental regulation. These three criteria together imply the need for diversity in delivery arrangements. However, analysis of current proposals is difficult because most proposals do not contain definitive provisions in many critical areas (about half the blocks in the table contain question marks). Moreover, it may be necessary to solve such problems as delivery acceptability and cost efficiency by legislation other than national health insurance.

Cost of National Health Insurance

The cost of national health insurance cannot be estimated accurately at this time and estimates have varied considerably. For example, in 1970 Saul Waldman estimated the cost of the AMA tax incentive proposal at roughly $15 billion,[46] while Sylvester E. Berki (1972)[47] estimated the cost at $4 billion. The First National City Bank has estimated that with enactment of the Kennedy-Griffith's bill health care expenditures in 1975 would be 8.7 percent of Gross National Product compared with 8.3 percent if the Nixon proposal became law, and 7.9 percent if no national health insurance legislation were passed.[48]

Joseph Newhouse, Charles E. Phelps, and William Schwartz have estimated the cost of two alternative types of health insurance plans. The first would provide full coverage with no coinsurance while the second would require a 25 percent coinsurance rate. Under either plan there will probably be only a slight increase in demand for hospital services because present insurance coverage for such services is nearly universal. They estimate an increase in demand for hospital services of 5 to 15 percent with a full coverage plan and roughly 5 percent with the 25 percent coinsurance plan.[49]

There will be a large increase in demand under either plan for ambulatory services since present coverage is less than in the case of hospital insurance. Moreover, the elasticity of demand for ambulatory services is greater than for hospital services. Thus, Joseph Newhouse, et al., expect that a full coverage plan would induce a 75 percent increase in demand, and a 25 percent coinsurance provision would induce a 30 percent increase in demand for ambulatory services.[50]

Furthermore, they estimate that the dollar cost for hospital and ambulatory services combined would be from $8 to $16 billion for a full coverage plan and $3 to $7 billion for a 25 percent maximum coinsurance plan.

Small deductibles (for example, $100 or $150 per person per year) would have little effect on demand for hospital services, but they could exert an important effect on reducing demand for ambulatory services. Available data do not permit a quantitative estimate of the effect of small deductibles on the demand for ambulatory services.

Summary

The private health insurance industry has grown very rapidly since World War II and presently accounts for slightly over 40 percent of all health care expenditures. While 80 percent of the population have hospital insurance coverage, less than 9 percent have dental care insurance.

Health maintenance organizations provide comprehensive health care services under a prepaid fixed capitation arrangement. Limited evaluation of HMOs indicate that they result in reductions in the rate of hospitalization and concomitantly lower costs of medical care than conventional Blue Cross plans or commercial health insurance.

The provisions of a number of national health insurance proposals were reviewed in terms of the six criteria developed by Robert D. Eilers. While greater financial accessibility and consumer participation in cost were the two criteria most readily satisfied, an analysis of current proposals is difficult because many bills do not contain provisions with respect to a number of the enumerated criteria.

Recent work by Newhouse, et al., indicates that the dollar cost for hospital and ambulatory services together would range from $8 to $16 billion for a plan offering complete coverage while a 25 percent coinsurance plan would cost $3 to $7 billion.

Notes

1. Herbert E. Klarman, *The Economics of Health* (New York: Columbia University Press, 1965), p. 31.

2. Health Insurance Institute, *Source Book of Health Insurance Data, 1973-1974* (New York: Health Insurance Institute, 1974), p. 8.

3. Sylvia A. Law, *Blue Cross: What Went Wrong* (New Haven, Connecticut: Yale University Press, 1974), p. 11.

4. Law, *Blue Cross*, p. 12.

5. Marjorie S. Mueller, "Private Health Insurance in 1972: Health Care Services, Enrollment and Finances," *Social Security Bulletin*, Vol. 37, No. 2, February 1974, p. 31.

6. Mueller, "Private Health Insurance," p. 32.

7. Ibid.

8. James O. Hepner and Donna M. Hepner, *The Health Strategy Game: A Challenge for Reorganization and Management* (St. Louis: The C.V. Mosby Co., 1973), p. 275.

9. William R. Roy, *The Proposed Health Maintenance Organization Act of 1972* (Washington, D.C.: Science and Health Communications Group, 1972), p. 13.

10. Charles G. Oakes, *The Walking Patient and the Health Crisis* (Columbia, South Carolina: University of South Carolina Press, 1973), p. 239.

11. Malcolm Peterson, "The First Year in Columbia: Assessments of Low Hospitalization and High Office Use," *Johns Hopkins Medical Journal*, Vol. 128, January 1971, p. 18.

12. Milton I. Roemer, Robert W. Hetherington, Carl E. Hopkins, Arthur E. Gerst, Eleanor Parsons, and Donald M. Long, *Health Insurance Effects: Services, Expenditures and Attitudes Under Three Types of Plan* (Ann Arbor, Michigan: University of Michigan School of Public Health, 1972), p. 34.

13. Joel Kovner, L. Brian Browne, and Arnold I. Kisch, "Income and Use of Outpatient Medical Care by the Insured," *Inquiry*, Vol. 6, June 1969, p. 33.

14. Roemer, et al., *Health Insurance Effects*, pp. 44 and 49.

15. Milton I. Roemer and William Shonick, "HMO Performance: The Recent Evidence," *The Milbank Memorial Fund Quarterly*, Vol. 51, No. 3, Summer, 1973, p. 294.

16. Robert L. Robertson, "Economic Effect of Personal Health Services: Work Loss in a Public School Teacher Population," *American Journal of Public Health*, Vol. 61, January 1971, p. 35.

17. Mueller, "Private Health Insurance," p. 22.

18. Health Insurance Institute of America, "Prepaid Group Practice and HMO's' Present Degree of Insurance Company Involvement in HMO Developments as of February 1, 1973," *Medical Economics Bulletin*, No. 4.

19. Program Status as of December 1972, Health Services and Mental Health Administration, Health Maintenance Organization Service, March 1973.

20. *American Medical News*, February 25, 1974, p. 9.

21. Oakes, *The Walking Patient*, p. 92.

22. Hepner and Hepner, *The Health Strategy Game*, p. 272.

23. U.S. Department of Health, Education and Welfare, *Report of the National Advisory Commission on Health Manpower*, Vol. II, Appendix 4, "The Kaiser Foundation Medical Care Program" (Washington, D.C.: U.S. Government Printing Office, 1967), p. 214.

24. For a discussion of this, see Odin Anderson, et al., *Comprehensive Medical Insurance* (Chicago, Illinois: University of Chicago, Health Information Foundation Research Series, 1959), No. 9, p. 11.

25. Paul Densen, et al., "Prepaid Medical Care and Hospital Utilization in a Dual Choice Situation," *American Journal of Public Health*, Vol. 50, No. 11, November 1960, p. 1710.

26. Densen, "Prepaid Medical Care," p. 1713.

27. John M. Glasgow, "Prepaid Group Practice as a National Health Policy: Problems and Perspectives," *Inquiry*, Vol. 9, No. 1, March 1972, pp. 4-5.

28. Avedis Donabedian, "An Evaluation of Prepaid Group Practice," *Inquiry*, Vol. 6, September 1969, p. 10.

29. *Journal of the American Medical Association*, October 30, 1951, p. 1560, quoted in Elton Rayack, *Professional Power and American Medicine* (Cleveland, Ohio: World Publishing Co., 1967), p. 138.

30. Sylvester E. Berki, "National Health Insurance: An Idea Whose Time Has Come," *The Annals of the American Academy of Political and Social Science*, Vol. 399, January 1972, p. 127.

31. Eveline M. Burns, *Health Services for Tomorrow: Trends and Issues* (New York: Dunellen, 1973), p. 145.

32. *Medical Care for the American People*, Final Report of the Committee on the Costs of Medical Care (adopted October 31, 1932). Reprinted U.S. Department of Health, Education and Welfare, 1970, Public Health Service (Washington, D.C.: U.S. Government Printing Office), p. 164.

33. Herman M. Somers and Anne R. Somers, *Medicare and the Hospitals: Issues and Prospects* (Washington, D.C.: The Brookings Institution, 1967), p. 5.

34. Saul Waldman, *National Health Insurance Proposals: Provisions of Bills Introduced in the 93rd Congress as of February 1974* (Washington, D.C.: U.S. Government Printing Office, 1974), Department of Health, Education and Welfare Publication (SSA) 11920.

35. U.S. Department of Health, Education and Welfare, *Expenditures for Personal Health Services: National Trends and Variations, 1953-1970* (Washington, D.C.: U.S. Government Printing Office, 1974), Publication No. 74-3105, p. 8.

36. Robert D. Eilers and Sue S. Moyerman (Eds.), *National Health Insurance Conference Proceedings* (Homewood, Illinois: Richard D. Irwin, 1971), p. 2.

37. Robert D. Eilers, "National Health Insurance: What Kind and How Much," (Part I), *New England Journal of Medicine*, Vol. 284, No. 16, April 22, 1971, pp. 883-86.

38. Eilers, "National Health Insurance," p. 883.

39. Ibid., p. 884.

40. Ibid., p. 886.

41. Robert D. Eilers, "National Health Insurance: What Kind and How Much," (Part II), *New England Journal of Medicine*, Vol. 284, No. 17, April 29, 1971, p. 950.

42. John Brittain, *The Payroll Tax for Social Security* (Washington, D.C.: The Brookings Institution, 1973).

43. Rashi Fein, "The Nixon Prescription for Health Care," *Washington Post*, March 10, 1974, p. B-1.

44. Fein, "The Nixon Prescription," p. B-5.

45. M.S. Feldstein, "National Health Insurance—A New Approach," Discussion Paper No. 150, Harvard Institute of Economic Research, November 1970.

46. Saul Waldman, "Tax Credits for Private Health Insurance: Cost Estimates for Alternative Proposals for 1970," *Medical Care*, September-October 1970, Vol. 8, No. 5, p. 365.

47. Berki, "National Health Insurance," p. 139.

48. First National City Bank, "Health Insurance—Getting the Prescription Right," October 1974, p. 14.

49. Joseph Newhouse, Charles E. Phelps, and William Schwartz, *Policy Options and the Impact of National Health Insurance*, R-1528-HEW/OEO (Santa Monica, California: Rand Corporation, June 1974), p. v.

50. Ibid.

Index

195